Inequality and Old Age

Inequality and Old Age

John A. Vincent
University of Exeter

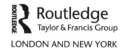

Routledge
Taylor & Francis Group

LONDON AND NEW YORK

First published in 1995 by UCL Press

Reprinted 2003 by Routledge
11 New Fetter Lane
London, EC4P 4EE

Routledge is an imprint of the
Taylor & Francis Group

British Library Cataloguing in Publication Data
A catalogue record for this book is available from the British Library.

ISBNs
1-85728-262-0 HB
1-85728-263-9 PB

Printed and Bound by Antony Rowe Ltd., Eastbourne, East Sussex.

Contents

Acknowledgements

I should like to gratefully acknowledge the assistance of a great many people in preparing this book, especially Rob Ashmore, Barry Barnes, Pam Barnes, Mary Guy, Paul Keating, Sue Milward, Zeljka Mudrovcic, Alison Tupman, Jamie Vincent, Sarah Vincent, Ros Weber and others. I also acknowledge the help of the ESRC Data Archive, and the Manchester Computing Centre, for the use of the General Household Survey and Family Expenditure Survey. The final result, and its limitations, are of course my responsibility alone. Many elderly people across the world took the time and trouble to talk to me, for which I am very grateful. In particular, I should like to remember those many people in Bosnia – where I worked on the first draft of this book – who helped me most generously before their country was torn apart by invasion, terror and international toleration of genocide.

Introduction

This book was written for both personal and professional reasons. The personal reason began when I became fascinated listening to old people and their accounts of their lives and the history of their communities. I enjoyed listening to my grandmother and other elderly relatives. Then, as a professional community worker and volunteer, I was involved with visiting elderly people and setting up services with them. I gained an insight into my family's history and could locate this in the social changes of the last one hundred and twenty years: in the rural-urban migration of skilled artisans to London, and in the subsequent expansion and suburbanization of London. An insight into changes in the British working-class movement came, not from books, but from the recollections of participants whose names would never reach the history books. Being involved in local government as an elected councillor and trying to provide improved services for elderly people led me to realize the extent to which problems concerning elderly people in our society are little understood and under-researched, and I was able to turn this into a systematic academic study. Finally, my position as a university lecturer, my training as a social anthropologist and my knowledge as a sociologist enabled me to attempt this study, for my growing personal interest coincided with a more general growth of interest in the subject and an increasing demand for research in the field, which clearly coincides with demographic changes in our society and across the world.

In this book, I shall attempt a sociological analysis of inequality by examining the issue of old age. This examination will cover the social processes in our society whereby age has become more important than it was in the past, and also how in contemporary society people experience old age as adversely affecting their social position. The purpose of this book is not to provide detailed figures for the percentages of elderly people who are fit, or who need medical care, or meals on wheels as most old people are fit, do not require medical care or social support and are as diverse a set of people as can be found within any other social category in society. Rather, by using anthropological and sociological analysis, it is my intention to provide some insight into the causes of these contemporary changes in the social position of elderly people. A better understanding of how the current social position of elderly people comes about may suggest ways in which we may achieve valued status in the final third of our lives. The key issues tackled in this book are about both social structure and moral values: that is, I ask not only "How do elderly people fit into society?", but also "What value should society attach to them?"

The original contribution of the book lies in drawing on a broad range of social science literature and linking this to issues of inequality and old age. These sources include social anthropology – to give a broad cross-cultural basis to the argument – British and American social gerontology, some social theory, some social policy and some historical material. I will also make use of original material from my own fieldwork in Italy, Ireland and Bosnia. The key concepts that provide intellectual integration to the book are those of the life course and of structured dependency. I discuss the original use of these terms and how various writers have tried to develop and extend them. The ideas allow a reconceptualization of inequality as a feature of life courses, rather than as a characteristic of some simple, abstracted, atemporal idea of an individual. The broader idea of structured dependency allows us to see the social processes by which power is exercised to generate inequality. In elucidating these processes of power it is possible to incorporate age as well as class, race and gender into a more general understanding of how it is that we live in an unequal society. The specific theoretical problem that the book seeks to address is why, in modern Western societies, elderly people have such an unequal position compared to those who, by virtue of their age, are considered to be in "the prime of their lives". Not all old people are powerless and dependent but all seem to undergo some experience of *social* devaluation at the end of the life course. What is the nature of this relationship of old age to inequality?

There is a particular need to consider these issues of old age and inequality at the moment; first, because elderly people are being labelled as a problem, apparently because there are more of them; secondly, because I see contemporary sociology losing its ability to comment critically on the condition of society and its collective inequalities, including that of old age. Furthermore, the importance of the topic is not restricted to people who are themselves in, or approaching, later life. The condition of older people is being constructed as a social problem and some sections of society are seeking to label social and demographic changes, involving increased numbers of elderly people, as a crisis. The press have started to pick up themes that are reflected in headlines such as "Britain bracing for the age bomb" (*Independent on Sunday* 29 March 1992), "State pension for all 'may have to go'" (*Guardian* 8 April 1993). There are programmes in the media that reflect rising levels of interest and concern. These are not only documentaries on medical and welfare aspects of the lives of the elderly but also drama and light entertainment programmes. *The golden girls, Waiting for god*, and *One foot in the grave*, have all achieved significant levels of popularity in Britain. This growing interest is also reflected in a prestigious inquiry and attempt to put public discussion of the Third Age high on the public agenda (Carnegie Inquiry 1993). However, questions have to be asked about why issues around old age are now attracting greater public attention. Is it merely because of these demographic trends and the fact that there are greater numbers, and/or greater proportions of elderly people in many countries? Alternatively, is it to do with growing levels of inequality and broader social and political issues about the distribution of power and wealth in society?

There is a need within sociology itself that makes such a study as this timely. Issues about material inequalities should be returned to the heart of the subject. It has become dominated, in theoretical terms, by a woolly relativism that is fundamentally unable to offer a progressive critique of contemporary society. The collapse of the Soviet Union has undermined the credibility of materialist accounts of social progress, which, together with the failure of market models and radical individualism to solve the growing problems of Western and global societies, have led to a vacuum in progressive social theory. There is a great need for theory based on the collective nature of society and informed by an understanding of history, which can act as a tool that people can use to gain an insight into how to act to improve their society. I hope to make some contribution to the revitalization of theories of inequality. I believe this is possible through a holistic theory of inequality that can accommodate all inequality – not only class, or race, or gender, but also age – and is holistic in a further sense in that it takes into account complete persons, including all their life and experience in a historically changing context (i.e. their life course).

What is inequality?

It is important to make the distinction between social differentiation and social inequality. Social differences are those human attributes that carry social meaning. All people are unique individuals; yet out of all the infinite number of possible differences between people, some contrasts come to have a culturally defined meaning. That is, some human attributes are given social meaning and their presence or absence constitutes social difference. Social inequalities are a subset of social differences. Critics of the idea of equality from an economistic and radically individualistic point of view (Letwin 1983) should note that both difference and identity are socially constructed. The content and structure of possible social differentiation is extremely wide and only some social differences involve inequality. Inequality involves a moral judgement, an evaluation of a social difference as better or worse. If things are incommensurable they cannot be unequal. There must be some degree of social agreement on the scale of evaluation, for social inequality to operate. Moral judgements are, by their nature, social. It is possible to cite contrasting cross-cultural situations where the same item or action was assessed on similar scales but with reversed positive and negative poles. Take, for example, Aztec human sacrifice. From the believers' point of view, the more sacrifices the better; from another perspective, the more sacrifices the greater horror (Farb 1969: chap. 11). Similarly, different cultures may evaluate the same body shape either positively or negatively. In some cultures fatter bodies are considered better (Evans-Pritchard 1940), while in others social shame is attached to fat (Turner 1984). Inequality concerns the social differences that are recognized in society and that are given positive or negative value.

4

Social differences are not necessarily associated with greater or lesser social esteem but, of course, very many are. It is precisely this process, by which social attributes come to have meaning and a positive or a negative evaluation, that is the stuff of sociology. However, there is an important point to be made: that social differentiation requires a cultural system of classification (Durkheim & Mauss 1963). Cultures are systems of generalization: they allow us to understand the world by putting the impossibly large number of unique things we encounter into a limited number of comprehensible categories. However, not only are cultural categories differentiated by selected attributes but, by the same process, they may also be classed as the same. Social inequality and social stratification are more specific varieties of social difference. Further, these two concepts should be kept distinct: social stratification being the process by which *groups* of people in society become differentially evaluated; while social inequality may not necessarily be a group attribute, and indeed different attributes of the same individual may lead that person to be rated as high or low on different occasions and in different contexts. However, this analytical point should not disguise the fact that most societies, including current modern industrial societies, are characterized by systematic, society-wide inequalities that fundamentally structure people's lives. This book is concerned with those inequalities that underpin social stratification.

Systematic general inequalities are built into the structure of society, such that relationships between groups of people are produced and constantly reproduced through significant periods of time. Social inequality arises in a systematic way that is related to how powerful people and institutions act towards social difference. It follows that social inequalities are systematically related to the power structure of society. The process by which inequality is created and recreated through time produces an observable and consistent shape to social relationships. Such systematic inequalities are structured into various patterns that are usually referred to as social stratification. For example, elderly people receive, on average, less of that most desirable of social goods, a cash income, than do those in middle age. Powerful groups of people and institutions ensure that is the situation and that is how it remains. But of course they can always be opposed, and frequently are.

A key perspective of this book is that of historical sociology. It draws on theories that see society as a long-term unfolding process that involves both individual and collective action in ways that seek to avoid simplistic analytical priority being given to either free will or social determinism. One of the key arguments presented in the following pages is that the incorporation of the concept of life course can significantly strengthen social theory by providing an inter-mediate level of analysis to link dynamically historical trends of long duration with immediate, everyday personal experience. The concept of the life course provides a means of connecting key social processes: historical development and change; the patterns of cohort and generation; and the experiences and choices of individuals, and their personal development. Inequality needs to be understood on all these levels and the concept of the life course turns out to be particularly helpful in achieving this objective.

This book does not stand outside, but rather is an integral part of, the social process by which elderly people and others may under-stand and shape their lives. Moody (1992) has used the work of Habermas to strengthen and clarify the objectives of critical gerontol-ogy. The purpose of the theoretical discussions in this book is to gen-erate communicative understanding (Habermas 1984), rather than instrumental knowledge. I seek to communicate ideas and theories in ways that will assist us to understand ourselves somewhat better and, as a result, liberate ourselves from oppressions such as ageism, in life-enhancing ways. The ultimate success of this book should be judged in these terms.

Age strata, generation, cohort, life cycle and life course

Developing new perspectives on the subject of inequality and old age requires a tightening-up of certain definitions used in the study of the dynamics of old age. The key terms that need to be defined are: age strata, generation, cohort, life cycle and life course. The defini-tions should be judged by their practical utility in adequately linking issues of time, ageing, history and social reproduction, to theories of inequality, stratification and social process.

"Age strata" are groups of people of the same age who by virtue of this characteristic have similar social rights and duties, even though members of these strata may have life courses that differ. For example, all those in England over the age of 18 are free to marry without the permission of their parents. Age strata are sometimes also called age classes. These are groups of people of the same age who, as a result of their common age, have a distinctive set of life chances. The roles and norms society allocates to age groups create barriers and opportunities. This can be seen to give people of similar age common interests as against those of people of other chronological age. A weak view of age strata would be simply that they are people in the same chronological age band; a strong view would be that they are people who have conflictual common interests over and against other age classes. People will move in and out of age strata as they add years to their life. The point about age classes in modern societies is that retirement (65 for men and 60 for women in Britain up until the legislation of 1994) is age specific – as are certain civil rights and responsibilities such as voting, marriage, sex, consumption of alcohol and tobacco, etc. It is important to note that the boundaries of the age categories are not fixed by any objective criteria, independent of society. The age categories thought up by demographers or legislators, for their convenience, are just as much social constructs as any reported sense of common identity among teenagers, pensioners, or the over-40s. Because of historical social change, the age at which individuals born at different times acquired these age-based rights and duties may have been different. The experience of a generation, or the common experience of those born at a particular time, can form part of developing age-based social structures.

"Generation" refers to the fact of reproduction and that each family experiences a sequence of people passing through the life cycle. Thus, today's children will be tomorrow's parents and will subsequently take their turn as grandparents. The use of the term "generation" can cause confusion. The idea of "age strata" is sometimes conflated with that of "generation". It is implied that the nation or the society is a family, such that those over 60 can be referred to as the "older generation". Similarly, "cohort" and "generation" are sometimes used in a potentially confusing manner; "the Sixties' generation" refers to people who were young during a particular period of history, i.e. to a particular cohort. The idea of "generation" can more usefully be restricted to refer specifically to a position within the family. Grandparenthood and retirement are not coterminous and neither are generation and age. Nephews and nieces may be older than their aunts or uncles, thus generation and age should also be rigorously distinguished conceptually.

"Cohorts" are sets of people born at the same time – thus, who age at the same time – and who, consequently, have many historical experiences in common. One view of historical social change is that of differing cohort experiences. Rapid change in society means that people with similar dates of birth may well have unique sets of experience. So, for example, the set of people in Britain who are in their eighties now were children in the First World War, were starting families in the Great Depression of the 1930s, went through the Second World War in prime middle age, and reached retirement when the post-war economic boom was stuttering to a close. These common experiences give that set of people a unique life course, and presumably a somewhat similar perception of the world, and so to some degree a sense of common identity. Similarly, it has been argued that the "generation" (correctly cohort) born in the post-war baby boom, who experienced the changes in social conventions of the 1960s and the collective sense of liberation at that time, consequently has a degree of common identity. One social repercussion of this differing cohort experience is sometimes referred to as a "generation gap". However, these cohort differences are not merely cultural; demographic change, and other changes in family structure, will mean that the experience of parenthood, and other intergenerational social relations, will change. The life course now, much more typically, will include the experience of being a grandparent in middle age and a great-grandparent in later life.

Studying cohorts then shares with age strata study, the problem of the arbitrariness of boundaries. Just as age since birth is a continuous and not a discrete variable, so dates of birth are only allocatable by the use of culturally constructed calendrical systems. Age strata and cohorts are two separate bases on which social life is patterned. The life-chances of someone of a particular age do not necessarily coincide either with generation or cohort experience. Additionally, there is a dynamic pattern by which the life courses of different cohorts affect one another. The cohort currently aged 70–80 who were born in the years 1910–20, have been affected by the struggles, often through trade unions, of the preceding generation that started British society down the road towards universal retirement pensions. The success of those struggles enabled this cohort to retire in greater security than their parents. Subsequently, they have been affected by the increasing proclivity of their children to separate and divorce, and thus obstructed in meeting some of the previously held expectations of grandparental relations.

The "life cycle" is seen as the typical sequence of age categories in a society. It is most frequently looked at in terms of the sequence of generations; as a continually turning wheel. Thus, all members of society are thought to age by following typical sequences of roles, for example child, adolescent, spouse, parent, grandparent, then ancestor. "Life courses" are different, although naturally they are structured by life cycles. "Life cycle" is a static image of an unchanging society; "life course" is an image that reflects the flow of time and the sequencing of cohorts as well as generations. "Life courses" happen to people in historical time and in particular places, so they reflect the fact that "life cycles" change over time and place. "Life courses" vary not only between different social groups, for example across genders, but significantly they also vary historically.

The "life course" is the individual experience of the collective social process of ageing. Life courses are social because they have general and observable patterns, which are part of the structure of society. Life courses can be seen to be structured by norms and values, for example those associated with the life cycle, but they are also given characteristic forms by historical patterns of social change. Thus, the life course is the normatively expected transition of stages in the process of social ageing and also, at the same time, reflects how such transitions themselves change. Hence the life course is both an individual and a social process of ageing. An individual's unique experience of life from birth (perhaps even conception) through to death (or at least the present) constitutes his or her life course. Life courses are sociological phenomena because experience through life is socially structured. They are periodicized through age strata sequences; the teenagers of today will become the pensioners of the next century. It is structured by the sequence of generations; today's children are tomorrow's great-grandparents. They are further structured by history, in that the life course of each succeeding cohort takes its form from the historical events through which it lives. The idea of the life course, in addition to these social and historical aspects, has a psychological dimension in that individuals will develop and change personality in response to life experience. Sometimes it is useful to refer to the individual life course as a life history (or possibly "career") to distinguish it from the generality of social processes and collective values that generate typical life courses. Kohli makes the analogy between base and superstructure on the one hand and hardware and software on the other (Kohli 1990). This

9

analogy identifies the life course as a set of basic parameters but individual lives as unique experiences, lived through the working-out of individual actions and social processes.

The life-course perspective has led to the development of new research methodologies. Empirical research using a life-course perspective requires studies of a longitudinal nature. There are strong professional, academic and social barriers to such research. The professional structure of academic life, including career prospects for researchers and identifiable results for funding agencies, militates against longitudinal study. Nevertheless, longitudinal studies over relatively short periods of less than a decade can produce significant results (Wenger 1986, 1990). The growing interest in life-history research reflects the evolving theoretical interest in the life course. Excellent quantitative investigations such as the Berlin Ageing Study into the condition of elderly people are constructed on such a theoretical base (Baltes et al. 1993). Qualitative methods for looking at how respondents reconstruct their life course in the process of telling it to the researcher are essential for those research strategies that rely on informants recounting life histories or recalling sequences of events (Bytheway 1989, Coleman 1991, Dex 1991, Samuel & Thompson 1990, Spenser 1990, Thompson et al. 1990). These methods tend to be both actor centred and critical of the limitations of "snapshot" surveys that tend to ignore cohort effects. The life-history approach adopted by many writers enables the significance of social and personal change to be studied from the point of view of elderly people themselves (Johnson 1978). Historical data and an understanding of changing historical conditions, within which to locate emerging life-course patterns, are also essential for contextualizing life-history studies. Examples of this approach are the work of Hareven (1982) in her study of New England immigrant workers over three generations, and that of Cribier (1989) in her study of the different experiences of different cohorts of Parisian pensioners.

In particular, the historical demography school, which has flourished at Cambridge, has developed techniques of using sources such as parish records to achieve detailed mapping of life-course events in historical populations (Laslett 1968, Laslett & Wall 1972, Watcher et al. 1978). The work of Peter Laslett is a good example of this type of study, and he has been led from this work to consider the social position of elderly people in contemporary society, and to try and change it. His work on the Third Age is extremely relevant to the issues discussed in this book (Laslett 1989). Peter Laslett has also engaged with an American-based set of literature, deriving from a combination of welfare economics and moral philosophy. This is the literature on the issue of "generational equity" (Laslett & Fishkin 1992). The originality of this approach to social justice and social policy lies in moving away from a "snapshot" view of society, and attempting to conceptualize social relationships across multiple generations. A number of writers in America, broadly under the headings of critical gerontology and moral economy, have developed a powerful critique of the inequalities experienced by elderly people. They have been significant participants in what has become known as the "generation equity" debate (Moody 1992, Minkler & Estes 1991, Cole 1993). I shall draw heavily on their work.

The structure of this book

This volume consists of an introduction and eight chapters. In Chapter 1, the nature of the issues under discussion is stated and it is established that old age can be considered as a source of social inequality, independent of biology or other sources of inequality. This chapter distinguishes the problem of inequality in old age from a range of other issues. It demonstrates that old age is not merely a biological problem but that it forms a cultural category crucial to the social analysis of inequality. The purpose of this chapter is to demarcate a topic area that is centrally located in sociology and a valid topic in social theory, namely inequality and old age, and demonstrates empirically the generality of disadvantage experienced by elderly people in modern society.

Chapter 2 examines the varieties of ways in which it is possible to be an elderly person across a wide range of societies. Old age has different effects and consequences in different societies, and life courses in each are subject to social change and variety, and this is demonstrated by drawing on a range of anthropological sources. These studies show that low social status in old age is far from inevitable. The chapter seeks to give some tentative explanations of the variety of statuses associated with elderly people.

Particularly significant is Chapter 3 because it introduces the life-course perspective. This perspective can be used to understand the position of elderly people in modern society and particularly how that condition has changed. This life-course perspective is especially useful in linking patterns of historical social change to the experience and activities of contemporary groups and individuals. Changing life-course patterns, including work careers and family career, are particularly significant in understanding the lifestyles of elderly people and the processes that lead to inequality. It is through the development of modern capitalist society and the values that accompany it that inequality for elderly people develops.

Chapter 4 attempts a cultural analysis of the meaning of old age. By drawing on linguistic manifestations of how old age is culturally constructed, and comparing the alternative ways in which it is elaborated and given meaning, it is possible to gain insights into the negative cultural image of old age in contemporary Western society. The symbolism of old age inevitably relates to the meaning given to death, and the chapter explores the links between the problems for Western society in comprehending death, and the social position it ascribes to elderly people.

These first four chapters establish that inequality in old age exists, that it can be the subject of social analysis, that it has a material and a cultural basis, and that it is subject to a very wide cross-cultural variation. One task of this book is to ask whether a non-ageist society is possible. However, to answer that question we must first have the necessary insights into how social inequality arises and changes. The second section of the book, which consists of a further four chapters, seeks to provide a new theoretical formulation of the issue of old age and inequality by providing a critique of some existing ideas and developing a new framework around inequalities of life course.

Chapter 5 presents a critique of existing approaches to inequalities of gender, ethnicity, class and age, and identifies those elements that are useful in comprehending age-based inequalities. This chapter takes the first steps towards a synthesis, by tackling the problem of material inequality in old age, and by seeking to locate elderly people in a general pattern that can provide an account of "who gets what" in modern capitalist societies.

The arguments that have sought to identify elderly people as a problem for society because of the interrelationships between demography and the provision of welfare and pensions are examined in Chapter 6. The chapter criticizes the suggestion that elderly people in the current generation will benefit at the expense of younger people.

The concept of generational equity is examined and used to demonstrate that a proper conceptualization of the relationships between generations can give a broader insight into the issue of inequality.

Chapter 7 looks at existing social theories of ageing that have not, on the whole, addressed the issue of inequality directly, to see what might be drawn from these sources for a more general theory of inequality. In particular by reassessing the political economy of old age and the concept of structured dependency, it is possible to identify useful parallels between the inequalities in old age and other systematically disadvantaged groups.

The concluding chapter, Chapter 8, seeks to make notes towards the construction of a theory of inequality. A generalized view of the nature of inequality is established. This is achieved by linking, on the one hand, cultural processes that lead to the social construction of difference and develop into ideological mechanisms for differential evaluation of social statuses; with a materialist account of power and domination, placing particular emphasis on expanding the idea of structured dependency, on the other. A crucial, dynamic element is added to the consideration of inequality on the basis of a life-course perspective. This final chapter argues that by considering the processes of inequality from a life-course perspective, it is possible to understand the relationship between class, race, gender and age as inequalities that are the product of common historical processes. From such a perspective it is possible to reconstruct a view of society in which there is potential for people – working class, black, female, elderly – to develop. It provides a tool that may help in the construction of a meaningful and positive role by elderly people for themselves in a changing society. By using the life course to link historical social forces to personal social action, inequality can be placed in a moral context, and the critical power of the ideal of equality does not become dissipated through fragmentation into a multitude of separate inequalities.

CHAPTER ONE

Social inequality and the ageing process

The purpose of this chapter is to establish that the study of inequality and old age is a real subject capable of being subjected to social scientific analysis. It will assert that there is a distinctive sociological study of old age, ageing and inequality, and further, although such study is related to the biological subject of gerontology, that there is a distinctive social science subject independent from it. Biological processes are significant for understanding the condition of elderly people, but overdeterministic assumptions about the universality and inevitability of poor health and low status in old age are misleading. The chapter goes on to consider whether there is a distinctive inequality associated with old age in modern Western society, which is independent of other forms of inequality.

Biological ageing

The first step is to discuss the relationship of the sociological and anthropological study of ageing and old age with that of biology and, more specifically, human physiology. What are the causes of ageing? What is meant by ageing as a natural process? Any living organism has a developmental pattern of physiological change that takes place over time, and that can be described as ageing. Human beings are no exception. The statement that we are dying from the moment that we are born is merely a reiteration of the finite life span available to the human species. Furthermore, over any life span, there are general patterns of observable change in human bodies. Obvious features of our bodies that change with age include, for example, the manifestations of sexual maturity through puberty, the menopause, and skeletal changes in later life (Bromley 1988, Gingold 1992).

Although there has been much research into the biology of ageing, there is still no universally accepted biological theory of ageing. There are basically two theoretical approaches to understanding why organisms age. The first is the "wear and tear" argument, which simply means that ageing is the process of the body wearing out. The second, alternative approach, suggests there is a kind of biological time clock; that the alarm is set for a certain time span and that the body will switch itself off when the alarm goes. Using an alternative analogy, this theory suggests that the body has a system of planned obsolescence. There are various mechanisms that are thought to play a role in biological ageing. The auto-immune theory suggests that the immune system becomes less effective with age; that the body's ability to deal with the things that cause death, such as infection, works less well. Of course, people die of something. They do not die of old age – they die because their heart stops beating, or because their brain ceases to function, or from some other direct biological failure of the body to sustain itself. A further feature of ageing is the loss of connective tissue, collagen. This is the feature that leads to the wrinkled appearance of older people. Theories that emphasize these and similar changes suggest, in essence, that the efficiency of the body in co-ordinating its different parts and having them work together ceases to operate properly. These views could be associated with the "wear and tear" argument. The "biological time clock" perspective links to the idea of cellular ageing. Over a life-time the actual molecular constituents of the body are replaced many times. Cells replace themselves by division and the idea is that there are a finite number of cell divisions possible after which the cells become too old to reproduce themselves properly and the life span has been completed. Advances in genetics that enable the identification of characteristics with particular genes, as exemplified by the human genome project, have boosted the view that the "human time clock" has a genetic basis. One recent popularization of this genetic approach under the title "suicidal cells" suggested that all cells had a tendency to self-destruct, which was counteracted by a specific, genetically controlled, biochemical process. It is the genetically timed removal of this

16

protective mechanism that is seen to lead to ageing and death (Hooyman & Kiyak 1988, Briggs 1990, Mayer 1987).

When ageing is seen as a post-maturity phenomenon, it is associated with a gradually diminishing rate of efficiency of the body (Spencer 1990). There is, however, considerable variation in human ageing and even within the same individual, organs do not all age at the same rate. Although some slowing-down of bodily function in old age seems inevitable, it can be controlled or retarded through appropriate behaviour including proper exercise, appropriate nutrition and similar measures. Factors through life, particularly work environments, nutritional regimes, trauma, etc. influence health in later life. For example, there is an association between age and hearing, and men are more likely to suffer hearing loss than women. There may be biological reasons for this, but there are clearly also social and environmental reasons (such as working with printing presses, pneumatic drills, etc.) why, on average, men's working lives have been more likely to expose them to the kinds of situation that are damaging to hearing. Social and environmental stress play an incompletely understood role in the development of disease and ageing. In practice, ageing is a complex interplay between social and biological processes. The assumption that biological ageing is a direct and universal process needs to be modified.

The interrelationship of the biological and the social

The biology of ageing is not irrelevant to the social inequalities associated with old age, but the relationship is far from direct. For example, gender inequalities vary over the life cycle in many societies. Sex-based roles tend to have less social salience at the beginning and end of life when sexual, and in particular, reproductive activity is less likely. This relationship seems to be widespread across the world, independent of the specific degree of gender inequality encountered in a particular society (Arber & Ginn 1991, Sanday 1981, Turnball 1984, Sharma 1980). This is not to argue that the biology of reproduction "causes" this social pattern. In Western society the bodies of the very young and the very old are open to touch, control and discipline by others in ways in which the bodies of those in their "prime" are not. Nappies are changed, noses wiped, incontinence pads changed; the very young and the very old are the object of washing behaviour decided upon and performed by others. The genders at either end of the life cycle are more nearly equal in their low status as "young" or "old" than they are in the fully adult stages of life.

Biological processes such as birth and maturation require a societal response. One such response is often called socialization, and includes methods by which the control of bodily functions are taught and learnt. Similarly, the biological processes of ageing and death require a societal response if society is to continue to function. Such functional prerequisites, however, are not highly determined in that social life is so flexible there are more social responses possible than our culturally bound imaginations can conceptualize. I am not advancing a teleological argument, that the social phenomena of age-based roles are caused by society's need to deal with death and ageing. Rather, there is a biological framework − for example the human life span − which, at a very general level, creates an opportunity structure within which human societies can develop. There is no simple determining relationship between biological ageing and social behaviour.

Age-related competences illustrate the nature of this biological base. During the process of maturation children learn some skills before others, and there is an identifiable, mean age by which certain skills, such as language acquisition, usually occur. However, some children can learn some skills at an earlier age than others and there is a wide range of variation in aptitude for one skill as opposed to another. But, most significantly, the specific skills learnt are infinitely socially variable; which language is learnt, who acquires which skills and how these abilities are all socially enacted. How much of the human biological potential is developed, and in what manner, is a product of society.

The idea of the life course is a concept that is particularly useful in combining social and individual perspectives (Harris 1987). Contemporary individuals' experience of old age is framed by both their individual age and position along a biological life span and also by the demographic structure of society. The latter, the emerging demographic profile of society, is of course the pattern that shapes the contemporary distribution of life courses. It is possible to illustrate this point at a simplistic level by pointing out that, given the pattern of human female biological maturation, development and ageing (i.e. the typical individual biological life course), there is a finite number of generations that can possibly be living at any one time, approximately six. Yet social constraints, in fact, tend to limit them still further. These social factors also affect demographic patterns of natality, mortality and migration. These will determine the size of the various living generations and thus affect the life-course experience of any individual (at least in terms of relationships with other generations). Thus at a very basic level, biology sets the framework in which the social relationship between generations can develop. But it can be seen that the biological framework does not set a tight limitation on social relationships and thus the most interesting questions about inequality between age groups and generations cannot be answered from the perspective of human biology.

The relationship between the biological and the social is not static, nor does it flow in one direction. There is a dynamic, reciprocal relationship between the social and the biological, because not only does the biology of individuals or a population place constraints on their possible social activities, but also, reciprocally, social activities influence people's biology. Sexual activity in old age is as much to do with the social availability of partners as with the ageing of the biological apparatus. Social behaviour and personality have physiological effects. The way people live affects the way they age and die. For example, the social influences summarized as social class, ethnicity or rural/urban lifestyles are associated with variations in the behaviour and health of elderly people. These effects can be noted in indicators of longevity. People's health in later life is related, among other things, to the kinds of work experience they have had through their life-time. At various times through life, nutrition shortfalls, exposure to stress and violence, and addictions (socially approved or not) can manifest themselves in behaviour patterns in old age (Riley et al. 1983, Palmore & Stone 1973). Marriage provides an obvious example of the impact of a social institution on longevity. Men have a shorter life expectancy than women. This is especially noticeable amongst men who live outside marriage through widowhood, divorce or bachelorhood. It is suggested that for both sexes marriage insulates against death, but this seems to be particularly true for men.

Age, ability and disability

There are particular patterns of symptoms and disease diagnoses associated with age. These include mobility-restricting handicaps such as rheumatism, arthritis, angina, etc. Frequent associations have also been made between age and changes in brain function leading to Alzheimer's disease, other forms of senile dementia and organically based mental illnesses such as some forms of depression. Not all old people will experience such problems but the prevalence of diagnosis of such disorders increases in older populations. I would not wish to reinforce the stereotype that elderly people are also disabled but there is an important link between discussions of old age and of disability. Elderly people are not necessarily disabled, but because some old people acquire specific disabilities during their lifetime they therefore experience similar social disadvantages to other disabled people. First, because elderly people are stereotyped as having disabilities and share with disabled people in general the disadvantages of a negative image, and secondly because both elderly and younger people experience their physical characteristics as abilities or disabilities on account of the nature of our society. It is important to be aware that most people labelled "disabled" are perfectly "able" in most aspects of their lives. However, their disability in one aspect often creates a stereotype, which is then carried through to other areas of ability. The title of the radio programme *Does he take sugar?* captures the way in which physical disability can be assumed to encompass mental limitations and lower social status. I can well recall my confusion and anger when, as a teenager, wheeling my father's wheelchair into a cinema, I was asked over his head whether he would like a smoking or non-smoking seat. At 13 it was difficult for me to comprehend why I was being asked to take responsibility for the prime authority figure in my life. Furthermore, someone missing a limb, or whose heart functions in a deviant way, is disabled only to the extent that society creates a physical and social environment that impairs such people's social performance. Those with dyslexia did not suffer disability in preliterate societies. Impairments such as limited vision that limit the ability to drive create "disability" in so far as public transport services are inadequate to meet people's transport needs. The disabilities of old age, just like other physical handicaps or abilities, are the result of an interplay between bodies and their capabilities and the functions society requires those bodies to perform.

20

Biological and demographic approaches to the study of ageing have different orientations with respect to the social nature of individuals. The human biology approach to ageing takes an individual perspective, in that the ageing individual is the subject of study, and there is an ideal typical model of an ageing body, pathologies being identified by deviation from the model. Demography, despite being based on certain individualistic assumptions, is about populations and looks at ageing from a societal perspective – the ageing process in this case is that of an ageing society. The sociological perspective tries to contain both individual and societal perspectives. It does this both by the study of meanings, *individuals* making sense of the world around them by using *socially* available meaning systems, and also by the study of institutions, *individuals* responding to the *social* roles available to them.

The sociology of age has shown that age is a socially manipulated category, the meaning of which is not determined by chronological age, or even by the biological process of maturation and ageing. In all societies, age is recognized as being of social significance. However, the meaning that is attributed and the roles that are allocated, or that are permissible, on the basis of age, vary enormously (Simmons 1970, Amoss & Harrell 1981). Sociology, being a critical discipline, is very reluctant to accept "natural" or common-sense statements at face value. Such statements are rather the objects of investigation. Thus a sociological question would be: How is it that some views of the world become unproblematic and apparently readily classify the great diversity of people into clearly explained types such that they appear to be common sense? The attributes of old age that are "obvious" can vary enormously from one culture to another, from "feeble-mindedness" to "wisdom", from "weakness" to "power". "In summary, Neugarten contends that chronological age simply does not correlate reliably with many socially important characteristics. It does not determine and hence does not predict attitudes, health, interests, education, family relationships, work capacity or intellect." (Nelson 1982: 144–5) This approach can form the basis for developing new attitudes and understanding towards elderly people. The removal of biological determinism allows us to understand the attributes of age just as we have come to understand gender and race: as a biologically based distinction that history and culture have exaggerated and elaborated into social roles to which older people are required to conform. Further, it enables us to see

21

that such conformity has come to be not only socially detrimental to elderly people but also culturally restrictive, and is a loss to society as a whole (Bytheway 1995). The sociology of age shows that there is no good reason to assume *a priori* that a chronologically old person is necessarily or significantly different in hopes, abilities and potential capacity from a chronologically middle-aged individual. Furthermore, it has identified government policies and cultural practices that impose and enforce such conformity as being arbitrary, discriminatory and potentially injurious to what is approaching a third of the population in modern Western societies (Neugarten 1982, McEwen 1990).

Is age an independent source of inequality?

A number of studies have helped to establish the extent of deprivation experienced by elderly people in Britain and America; in Britain, Townsend's work is an obvious example (Townsend 1957, 1979); as is that of Carroll Estes in America (Estes 1979, Estes et al. 1984, Estes & Minkler 1984, Estes & Swan 1993). Alan Walker has played a significant part in documenting the material disadvantages experienced by older people both in Britain and in Europe (Walker 1980, 1990a,b,c, 1993). Large-scale national surveys such as the Family Expenditure Survey and the General Household Survey can be used to illustrate the relationship of age to poverty. Some elderly people are rich and some poor, but the older the people are the more likely they are to be poor. Surveys of expenditure in the United Kingdom in 1991/2 showed men aged 60 years and over to have an average (median) net income per head, per week, of £108 compared to £173.70 for men aged 17–59. The equivalent figures for women are £58 and £80.59 respectively. However, for those aged over 74 years, income for men is down on average to £81.07 and for women it is £58.65 per week (General Household Survey 1991/2). The older group also has substantially reduced expenditure, compared to younger age groups, and there does seem to be potential for concern about a group of very poor elderly people whose standard of living is particularly vulnerable to a squeeze between the state pension and increases in the costs of gas, water, electricity and other basic essentials. The following figures (see Table 1.1) indicate not only the

Table 1.1 Average (median) normal weekly disposable household income by age.

| | Age of head of household | | | | Over |
	17–30	31–50	51–65	66–75	75
Household expenditure in £					
1985	168.33	237.97	206.77	130.82	88.20
1992	229.07	321.81	243.57	142.18	98.38
Expenditure per capita in £					
1985	69.18	71.37	87.85	75.08	62.78
1992	103.91	105.26	116.52	87.67	71.89

Source: Central Statistical Office, Family Expenditure Survey 1985 and 1992.

continuing relationship between age and financial wellbeing but also that, over a seven-year period of growing prosperity for many in Britain, the elderly population did not, on average, benefit as much as the middle aged.

After retirement, the inequalities resulting from low pay, unemployment, disability, ill health, sex discrimination and racial discrimination are carried through into old age. The decline in the value of savings and pensions, and cohort effects in development of pension systems, means the worst off are the very old. Data on earnings, income, assets, housing circumstances and benefits in kind, such as those recorded in the General Household Survey and other UK government large-scale surveys, indicate that the older old experience greater proportional poverty than the younger old who in turn have less than the national average (Johnson & Falkingham 1992: chap. 3). This may be due to cohort effects, as the greater prosperity during the life courses of the younger cohorts is reflected in such developments as occupational pensions, and contributes to the creation of age-based inequality (Baltes et al. 1993: 534). Nevertheless, the strong association of increasing age with increasing poverty is maintained across cohorts even though the absolute levels of deprivation might vary.

The low income of elderly people means that a large percentage of their expenditure goes on basic necessities. Among one- or two-pensioner households, food, housing and fuel takes an average 55.0% of expenditure. For the poorest 20 per cent of such households, it is 61.5% of expenditure (*Social Trends* 1989: 103). The equivalent figure for all households is 42.3% of expenditure. According to the 1992 Family Expenditure Survey, the average (mean) total weekly household expenditure for the country was £265.55, of which expenditure on food was 18% and on heat, light and fuel 5% (a combined figure of 23%). For the category of households whose household head was aged over 64, the survey reports an average weekly expenditure of £150.06 of which 22% went on food and 8% on heat, light and fuel (a total of 30%). For those in this elderly household category whose expenditure was under £50 per week the situation was even worse, with some 17% of expenditure going on heat, light and fuel, and over 50% of expenditure on this and food. For households with heads of household aged over 74 years, mean total weekly expenditure averaged at some £118.47 with 22% spent on food and 9% on heat, light and fuel (31% in all). A situation in which pensioners are spending such a high proportion of their outgoings on basic necessities suggests they are disadvantaged in the most fundamental material sense. The current controversies in Britain over the cost of basic necessities compared to pensions suggest that this is one vital source of the unequal position of the very old in British society.

The nationalized monopoly of power supplies in Britain enabled the government in the 1980s to impose what was effectively a gas tax. In equalizing prices between gas and electricity, gas bills to the consumer were forced up, and the excessive profits passed to the Exchequer. The lack of readily available alternative suppliers or sources of energy permits such clear "exploitation" (in the correct sense of the word) to occur. This source of economic power depends not just on the role of the state but on the "natural monopoly" of the supply of bulk domestic power and is unlikely to be alleviated by recent privatization in Britain of public gas and electricity utilities. Later, in the 1990s, a more direct attempt to raise revenue for the Exchequer by charging Value Added Tax on fuel, including gas, led to widespread public outcry and political opposition. This public controversy focused primarily on the position of elderly people who required warmth for survival and whose pensions would not increase by an equivalent amount.

The inequalities in the rest of society are reproduced in old age, and appear to be amplified. Inequalities of class interact with those of sex to produce a further strand of differentiation in old age. Two-thirds of pensioners are women, and in addition, 48 per cent of widows live at or below the Supplementary Benefit level (the poverty line in Britain) and women have the greater likelihood of being widowed. Women are also likely to live longer and the older old are those most likely to be poor (Arber & Ginn 1991). Victor and Evandrou's (1987) examination of the impact of class on old age reveals that the experience of old age is highly class specific and that class inequalities, rather than diminishing with age as is sometimes assumed, strongly determine the life-chances of elderly people. Furthermore, such inequalities are strongly influenced by housing tenure, which itself is strongly associated with class-based inequalities in lifestyle. People with non-manual occupations are more likely to have an occupational pension than those in manual jobs. The Royal Commission on the Distribution of Wealth while it was in operation reported that the average occupational pension for a professional or managerial worker in the Registrar General's class 1 was £20 per week while the equivalent figure for those in class 5, with unskilled manual jobs, was only £5 per week. In addition, white-collar workers are more likely to retire at the age of 60 and, given class-related distributions of health and morbidity, manual workers are less likely to have a complete contributions record for full pension rights and more likely to suffer from both physical and psychological illness. The absence of savings and a reasonable occupational pension means depending both upon state provision and on the state definition of what constitutes an acceptable old age (Evandrou & Victor 1989).

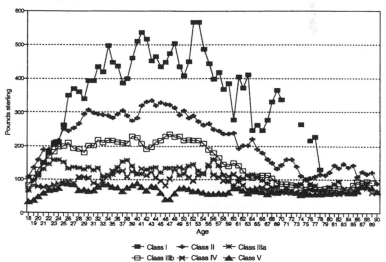

Figure 1.1 Median weekly income by age and class (three-year moving average). *Source:* author's analysis of General Household Survey 1991.

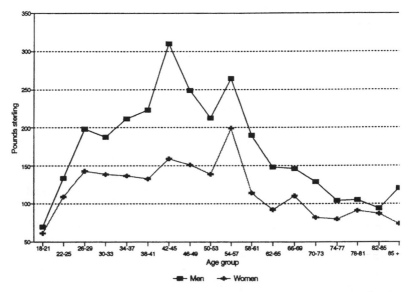

Figure 1.2 Median weekly income by age and gender. *Source:* author's analysis of General Household Survey 1991.

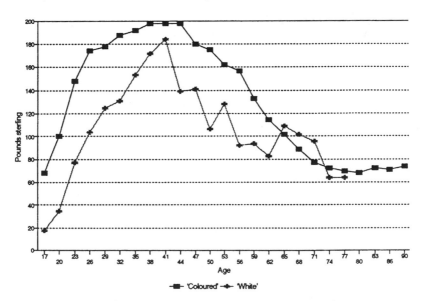

Figure 1.3 Median weekly income by age and race (three-year age bands). *Source:* author's analysis of General Household Survey 1991.

Figures 1.1, 1.2 and 1.3 indicate that there is a systematic curve that relates income to age. Income starts low, increases until middle age and declines through later years. This pattern has been around in Britain for at least a century, and has been called by some a "Rowntree-type cycle" after the classic study in York that identified the young and old as particularly vulnerable to poverty (Hedstrom & Ringen 1987, Rowntree 1901). This pattern is related to the employment patterns of modern society, and is visible across occupational groups and also clearly observable for women and for minorities (see Figs 1.1, 1.2 and 1.3).

It is also reported (Victor & Evandrou 1987) that the younger elderly are more likely to own a wide range of consumer durables than are the older elderly which is a further indication of the independent relationship of age to inequalities of lifestyle. Ownership of consumer durables indicates that both class and age are independently related to social inequality (see Table 1.2).

These figures suggest that semi-skilled and unskilled manual workers and their families in old age are systematically less likely than professional and managerial people of a similar age to own consumer durables considered appropriate to a modern lifestyle. However, those people over 75 in both class groups have less chance than their equivalents aged under 60 years of owning a phone, a freezer, central heating and other things that can make the lives of elderly people

Table 1.2 Ownership of consumer durables by age and occupation (in %).

	Colour TV	Phone	Central heating	Freezer	Video
Age 16–59					
Manager and professionals	97.6	97.3	93.3	93.3	88.3
White collar and skilled manual	95.7	88.1	81.7	88.0	83.4
Semi-skilled and unskilled	92.2	72.3	72.7	83.8	77.3
Age 60–74					
Manager and professionals	97.6	98.4	89.8	90.9	65.0
White collar and skilled manual	95.8	92.5	82.6	81.9	52.9
Semi-skilled and unskilled	91.3	83.7	78.8	71.2	46.9
Age 75 and over					
Manager and professionals	96.5	96.5	90.7	73.3	27.9
White collar and skilled manual	90.8	83.7	68.9	55.1	15.5
Semi-skilled and unskilled	88.8	77.2	67.9	47.5	8.6

Source: author's analysis of General Household Survey 1991.

Table 1.3 National differences in income and poverty by age.

	Disposable income in relation to national mean[1]			Poverty rates[2]		
	65–74	75+	All ages	65–74	75+	All ages
Canada	0.94	0.81	1.00	11.2	12.1	12.1
W. Germany	0.84	0.77	1.00	12.1	15.2	07.2
Israel	0.92	0.96	1.00	22.6	27.1	14.5
Norway	1.01	0.79	1.00	02.7	07.3	04.8
Sweden	0.96	0.78	1.00	00.0	00.0	05.0
UK	0.76	0.67	1.00	16.2	22.0	08.8
USA	0.99	0.84	1.00	17.8	25.5	16.9

1 Disposable income (adjusted for family size) as a proportion of the national mean for the total population.
2 Poverty rate defined as percentage of persons in families with adjusted disposable income below half of the median for all families in the population.
Source: Hedstrom & Ringen 1987 quoted in Walker 1990c.

more comfortable. The same trend, according to class and age, is evident for all five consumer durables considered in the table.

The pattern of inequality is found not only in Britain but also in the United States and widely across the industrialized world (see Table 1.3). Although some countries, particularly the Scandinavian welfare states, seem to be more effective in counteracting poverty in old age than others, the overarching trend is still visible. The basic pattern that, when you are past the "prime of life", the older you are the poorer on average you are likely to be is, although varying in extent and severity, maintained across the industrialized world.

Old people are, on average, poorer the older they become and this effect is independent of factors of sex, race and class (Cool 1987: 271). Working-class elderly people are on average poorer than the professional classes, elderly women are on average poorer than men, and black retirees poorer than white, but within each category increased age also brings increased poverty.

The age, sex and race gradients throughout Table 1.4 show how systematically older people as opposed to younger, women as opposed to men, and racial minorities as opposed to whites have lower incomes. The exception that proves the rule is the changed position of younger Hispanic elderly as opposed to the old when compared to the black groups. This feature must alert us to the importance of cohort effects and features such as the migration and employment histories of different groups of elderly people.

Table 1.4 Median income of persons aged 65 and older by age, race and sex in USA 1984 (in $).

Race	All races	White	Black	Hispanic
Both sexes				
65–69	8,250	8,655	5,431	5,033
70+	6,556	6,889	4,217	4,754
Male				
65–69	11,837	12,180	7,079	6,551
70+	8,663	9,109	5,114	5,289
Female				
65–69	5,782	5,966	4,477	4,289
70+	5,540	5,765	3,850	4,346

Source: Hooyman & Kiyak 1988: 404.

These data established that indicators of material wellbeing are systematically related to age. Further questions follow from this key observation: How do elderly people experience these inequalities? What divides elderly people and what do they have in common? The objective condition of inequality in which many elderly people live is experienced subjectively in a variety of ways. This subjective experience differs from many accounts of the social position of elderly people, including views from both left and right, presented by social scientists and other commentators. One of the specific intellectual problems that prompted this book was the view that pensioners were, through their receipt of pensions and benefits, consuming surplus value created by the productive sectors of society. Hence, presumably pensioners were "exploiting" those in work, in the technical sense of the word.

Is inequality a feature of age itself or merely of the cohort who are old at the present time? A frequent problem with gerontological studies is the cross-sectional fallacy (a comment that is also true in the broader context of sociological research). This cross-sectional fallacy derives from trying to explain the distribution of one variable (such as behaviour) from another (such as age) without regard to historically changing social circumstance. The older people are, the less likely they are to have experienced extended years of schooling or obtained certificates. No-one believes this relationship is causal, that old age is the cause of poor educational achievement. However, many appear to believe uncritically that the age correlation with loneliness, or some medical conditions, is a causal one (Riley et al. 1983). When the fallacious assumption of universal decline in old age is accepted unthinkingly in the sociological as well as popular literature, stereotypes that operate destructively as self-fulfilling prophecies are reinforced. Cohort centrism – seeing the world from the point of view of your own cohort, which, because of the social composition of the ranks of gerontologists, is usually that of middle-aged white males – is as limiting to clear vision as ethnocentrism, or phallocentrism (Riley 1988, Bytheway 1995).

How do the experiences through life of family, employment and other aspects of personal history relate to loss of status in old age? Does the loss of income and status occur simply as a result of age-based phenomena or does the common experience of a cohort separately form part of the developing structures associated with old age? There are demonstrable difficulties with the kind of approach that tabulates incomes and lifestyle variables in order to indicate systematic inequalities on the basis of age in our society. Riley (1988) argues that the apparent shift in the balance of resources from young to old age strata in recent years is the result of the distortions of the cross-section perspective. If the same issues of inequality and old age are looked at from a cohort perspective it can be shown that low status in youth and old age compared to middle age persists; the changes are merely that the old are entering old age in a richer and stronger position than previous cohorts. Riley goes further and speculates that if the depression and economic decline take a long-term hold and reverse the developments of modern times, the relationship of elderly people to those in middle age might change when the middle aged are no long better educated or, even, find themselves with fewer economic assets than members of older and richer cohorts (Riley 1988).

Surveys of current lifestyles of elderly people do not take sufficient account of cohort effects. Social studies that merely take a snapshot view of society are liable to produce distorted images and have profound limitations when identifying social processes. The response of social gerontologists to this critique has been to develop a life-course approach to the study of old age. The basic issue tackled in this book is how to explain the social inequality experienced by older people. This chapter has established that old age has a systematic impact on people's social condition, even when examined in conjunction with other social and biological variables. Women may be disadvantaged compared to men, but older women are disadvantaged compared to women as a whole. Similarly, working-class women are less equal to women as a whole in their material circumstances, but elderly working-class women are worse off still. What is it that systematically disadvantages older people? Individual attitudes and preferences cannot explain class effects on age or age effects on class; just as the increasing numbers of unemployed cannot be explained by a sudden upsurge in laziness. The features concerning age strata and cohorts that we have discussed in this section are structural features of society. The choices and opportunities of individuals are structured by the social groups of which they are a part and how these social groups fit together to make up society.

It is not satisfactory merely to develop an ever-growing shopping list of disadvantaged groups. Simply to add age to the triumvirate of class, race, and gender will not bring us closer to understanding social inequality (Bytheway 1995: 10). However, to integrate a satisfactory account of age-based inequalities with others would be to make progress. A theoretically adequate analysis of the inequalities associated with old age seems to me, therefore, a vital project at this time; not only to develop insights that will empower elderly people themselves, but, in doing so, to strengthen the analysis of social inequality as a whole. Ageing is a process by which all members of society have inequalities imposed on them; thus old age cross-cuts the categories of class, race and gender (Biggs 1993: 97–8). This is not to deny the powerful and cogent work that has demonstrated very great and growing inequalities between elderly people on the basis of class, race and gender (amongst others, Arber 1989, Arber & Ginn 1991, Estes et al. 1984, Blakemore & Boneham 1994). The point is, that within all these categories age is an effective way of creating disadvantage in advanced capitalist societies. What the male elderly and the female elderly have in common is that they are relatively more disadvantaged than their middle-aged counterparts. Similarly, it is not that the elderly are not profoundly divided by class and race, but that within racial and class categories those who are old experience relatively more deprivation.

CHAPTER TWO

Being old in different societies: varieties of ways to be an elderly person

The status of elderly people

This chapter takes a cross-cultural view of the inequalities associated with old age. It looks at the nature of, and theories about, the variations in the social status of elderly people in different societies. Just as the previous chapter showed that it is wrong to assume that for biological reasons elderly people, as they get older, decline in status, so this chapter seeks to demonstrate that there is broad variation in the social status of elderly people. There is no inevitable social process by which elderly people lose status. The decline in status is not assigned by the impersonal force of nature, but is a feature of particular societies and social processes. It is not universal and inevitable that old age is associated with poverty, loss of power and loss of status. In some societies old age leads to high social status and in some it leads to low. Although there are some universal features of biological ageing, which were discussed in the preceding chapter, the change in status associated with ageing is a social, not a biological, product. Is it possible to characterize the societies that are more likely to give high social status to the elderly, which hold them in esteem and give them social prestige? On the other hand, what characteristics will typify those societies in which old people have little or no power and little or no social honour?

The cross-cultural comparative method of anthropology can be particularly useful when dealing with large-scale issues of the human condition such as inequality (Farb 1969, Bodely 1983). It is particularly useful in overcoming the problems of ethnocentrism and the tendency to look at the problem through the blinkers of our own culture. It is one method that can be used to debate and expose the myths by which conventional inequalities and prejudices are explained and justified. By looking at a wide variety of different types of society that have been systematically documented by ethnographers, we can start to answer questions on status, old age and the life course. We can examine whether societies have a socially recognized category of "old people" (Ikels et al. 1992). We can look at how different cultures evaluate age and ageing, how they conceptualize the life course and its different elements, and make judgements about each part (Simmons 1970, Amoss & Harrell 1981).

I will present three examples from different kinds of societies. These societies are differentiated in terms of their mode of production: hunting and gathering societies; tribal (horticultural or pastoral) peoples; peasant cultivators. Of course by implication the comparison is also made with contemporary industrial societies such as Britain. These societies are shown within the anthropological convention of the "ethnographic present", that is to say they are described in a manner that refers to the social situation recorded by the anthropologists during the period they lived with the society. I will make use of studies of Tiwi gerontocracy (that is rule by the elderly) – the Tiwi are an Australian Aboriginal society. These societies were "band" societies in which characteristically, old age had high status, particularly for men. East African cattle herders, amongst others, are known for the social significance they attach to age grades and age sets. Peasant households across the world show a wide variety of forms and relationships, one of which is the patriarchal extended family. The relationship between age and family dynamics in peasant households will be illustrated with original ethnographic material from Val d'Aosta in northern Italy, and the Republic of Bosnia and Hercegovina.

We can start with some fairly simple propositions – generalizations that will have to be qualified and to which we must add concrete examples. In societies in which old people control valued rights, most notably those in property, land and women, old people are likely to have high status. This is also the case when they have valued rights because of their contacts with the supernatural. In societies that are based on lineal systems of kinship, the importance of elderly people as links in the chain of descent may give them status (La Fontaine 1978, Foner 1984, Silverman 1987a).

Tiwi gerontocracy

Let us first look at the Australian Aboriginal society, which was a hunting and gathering society without agriculture or pastoralism. People lived off the land, by collecting food directly from the environment. In this society kinship systems were highly elaborated and have been the fascination of anthropologists for generations. These societies have the characteristics of gerontocracies, in that elderly men dominate the political life of these societies and have the most power and status (cf. Berndt & Berndt 1983). Two anthropologists, Hart and Pilling, have provided us with an account of the Tiwi. Hart lived with the Tiwi in the period 1928–9 and Pilling during 1953–4, and in their book *The Tiwi of North Australia* (Hart & Pilling 1960) they describe how old people come to dominate this group. I will illustrate the process through an account of a dispute settling scene. This example is significant because it uses anthropological material to undercut Western preconceptions about human societies and ageist myths. It shows that, contrary to the noble savage image, violence does occur in such societies but, that in contrast to notions of the savage barbarian, such violence does not lead to the young fit men, the expected aggressors, dominating society. On the contrary, the younger men have to submit to the violence of the gerontocracy.

Conflict over women is fairly typical of materially simple societies who do not have property to accumulate and argue over. Tiwi bachelors were not able to acquire wives without the sponsorship of elderly men and then only after half a life-time of political manoeuvring to acquire their first wife in their late thirties and forties. Tiwi bachelors had to be satisfied with casual temporary liaisons and even these, if they came to light, were punished. Since senior men were able to dominate the marriage "market", they had young wives (wives who frequently had been betrothed at birth) and the young men were excluded. The seduction of a married woman was viewed as an offence by a young man against the husband and hence frequent charges were laid by senior men against younger. The most common accusation was a loud verbal complaint, for all the camp to hear, calling the young man to account for his actions. A public trial would result if the elder man wished to press the case, and would be held at a large public gathering. It took a standard form, which has been called a duel. Everyone present, including men, women and children, formed a rough circle with an open space in the middle. At

35

one end stood the accuser, the old man covered with white ceremonial paint with his spears in his hands, and at the opposite end of the arena stood the young man, with little or no paint and probably no weapon. The old man had not only ceremonial spears but also hunting spears, which were the effective ones in causing hurt. A weapon in the hands of the young man would be a sign of insolence, more likely he would only hold a throwing stick, which challenged the power and authority of the old man less blatantly. A proper sign of humility, which bachelors ought to show in this situation, would be to appear weaponless. The elderly accuser, with many dramatic gestures, elaborated to the young man and the community surrounding them precisely what he and all right-minded members of society thought of him and his misdemeanours. This loud harangue would go into minute detail not only of the accusation, but of the whole life history of the defendant, paying particular attention to occasions in the past when the elderly man or at least some of his relatives had performed some kindness to the young man or his relatives. The obvious function of this harangue was to remind the young man of his debt to society and re-establish proper social norms and to convey the idea that social life is mutual aid and trust between all its members, which such crimes as seduction would undermine. After an extended period of this abuse and blame-making, the old man would put aside his ceremonial spears and begin to throw his hunting spears at the young man. The protagonists were perhaps 10 feet apart and the young man would dodge and weave, without shifting his position in the arena too much, to avoid being hit by the spears. If the accused jumped too far out of the way he was jeered at; if the old man was wild, he also would attract some public ridicule. A fit young man would never be likely, except by miscalculation, to be hit by the spears of an old man. However, if he continued to dodge the spears for too long, the old man would look ridiculous, and old senior men should not look ridiculous in this society. Thus no young man who wished to become a respected elder himself would make such a challenge. The elders, after all, controlled access to marriage and women. Holding them up to public ridicule was certain to antagonize them all. So the young man, having demonstrated his physical ability, then showed a proper moral attitude by allowing himself to be hit. Trying to lose, without it being too obvious and without getting too badly injured, Hart and Pilling (1960) suggest, takes a skill of high order. When blood was shed, the crowd shouted with approval; the young man had behaved appropriately and the old man retrieved his honour, while the sanctity of marriage was upheld and everyone went home satisfied, full of moral rectitude – seduction did not pay (Hart & Pilling 1960: 81).

Some Tiwi young men did choose defiance, even though the dice were heavily loaded against them. There were various levels of defiance, the mildest being to refuse to let the old man's spears hit the target; rather more brazen was to turn up with a weapon and to brush aside the old man's spears. Such attempts to defy authority were met with a swift response. The duel, which began as two protagonists facing each other within a circle of spectators, would become one in which two or three or four old men would range themselves with their spears beside the accuser, against the culprit. Other old men would slowly leave their seats and conduct quiet diplomacy with the close relatives of the accused, particularly his brothers and his father, and gently lay restraining hands on them or lead them away. The young man was now facing the representatives of the gerontocracy without support: one spear could be escaped, but when a volley of spears came from the old man's allies they could not be avoided. This baring of society's teeth was usually enough for the younger man to submit, throw aside his weapons and be wounded. Continued defiance in the days before the Pax Australiana would have led to death (Hart & Pilling 1960: 82–3).

This example is significant for a number of further reasons. In addition to demonstrating that even in simple hunting and gathering societies older people could have power and prestige, it illustrates dramatic differences in the sequencing of the life course between men and women, sequences that show a marked contrast to our own society. For men, there is a prolonged period of bachelorhood. There is a long gap between initiation and being recognized as an adult member of society who can take responsibility for one's actions, and being a married man with the social status of head of a household unit and legitimate parent. Men have to wait until their late thirties to aspire to such roles. For women, on the other hand, this pattern of strategic and competitive marriage means being promised at birth to a marriage alliance. Women thus become fully functioning adult household members and parents at much younger ages than men. They outlive their husbands who may be thirty years their senior. These widows may still be fecund, and are still part of the marriage game. Older women, without fathers, and who lose their husbands, have a degree of status in negotiating their own marriage arrangements. Thus women as well as men in this society gain status with age. The social factors that enable this to happen are, first, a kinship system built around marriage alliance that places older people (particularly men) in a strategic position in society's social/kinship networks and thus gives them a degree of power over those not in such a strategic position (and who are younger). Further, power is reflected in the social allocation of scarce resources, in this case the sexual, economic, ritual and social status services that women provide. Control of these resources gives older people power and status. Thus in this society, the life course is structured in radically different ways for men and women, and the significant transitions that mark progress through life form significantly different sequences to those found in the contemporary West.

Age grades

Hunting and gathering societies are frequently made up of bands of 50–200 people, very simple in organization and with relationships on a personal level; thus, individual reputation is important to status. In more complex societies, associated with horticulture and pastoralism, it is more usual to find relationships based on kinship providing the structure to society. These societies are usually known as "tribal" societies in the literature of cultural evolution (White 1959, Sahlins 1968). However, many of these societies also use age as a method of social organization. Age sets are named social groups, age grades are social roles – functions specified for people of a certain socially defined age. Age sets are a formal institution, defined by initiation. They link together people of the same age across the whole society and thus integrate the different kinship groups together. Age sets produce a set of cross-cutting social ties that enable a greater degree of social integration and solidarity than would otherwise be achievable simply by the principles of descent. This grid effect enhances social solidarity, for example, in an environment where cattle raiding is endemic. This kind of organization is noticeably developed in the pastoral societies of East Africa. Well-known examples of these people are the Nuer (reported on by Evans-Pritchard in his classic study), the Karamjong, the Turkana, and the Masai (Evans-Pritchard 1940,

Bernardi 1985). A further example are the Samburu which are explicitly described by Spencer as a gerontocracy (Spencer 1965).

The Tiriki of Kenya illustrate age-group-based social organization (Sangree 1965). In this society, there are seven named age sets and each of these groups takes initiates – young men – over a fifteen-year period. There are parallel female institutions, but it is those for males that provide the public political framework of the society. A man becomes a man by going through an initiation ceremony with others. They join a particular age set, which is part of the fixed sequence of age sets that repeats itself about every 105 years. Thus the *Sawe* age set took initiates in the period 1843–58 and again between 1948 and 1963. When the age set is closed, a nationwide ceremony is held that marks the end of initiations into that age set and it is then said to "hold the land". All the other age sets move on to the next age grade, a particular set of roles in the age-based division of labour. The newly closed group is now in a position to make its name, to achieve a reputation that it will carry through the rest of its life. They are the warriors and in past times would raid and war as well as dance and womanize. When the next age set is closed, these warriors will become "elder warriors", the next age grade up. This is not as glamorous as the warrior group and the men of this grade begin to take administrative responsibilities and act as messengers. Men are also most likely to marry in this period. Judicial elders are those who take important administrative decisions, conduct arbitration, settle disputes, develop the policy of the tribe and are charged with promoting harmony within it. The oldest groups take on the function of ritual elders with a priestly function at ancestral shrines. They expel witches and conduct sorcery on behalf of the tribe. At the very oldest ages, the boundaries between age groups become less visible, although still of significance to the few remaining individuals. In independent Kenya, the Tiriki are part of a nation state, so the political functions of the age grades become less, the warriors cannot legitimately make war. But Sangree reports that the ceremonies continue and the ritual elders are universally feared and respected (Sangree 1965: 72).

In these kinds of societies, all men, provided they survive, can expect to reach positions of power and authority with advancing years. Although, of course, because of other factors such as size of herds, size of families, and personality traits, there will be differences between age-grade members, the basic social role is attained by all. It is a feature of these societies that they are what is called in the anthropological literature "acephalous" – literally headless. They do not have chiefs or pyramidal structures of authority, and in this respect they reflect the pastoral mode of production in which people are dispersed widely with their herds and where the possibility of central control is difficult (Weissleder 1978).

The functional explanation for the use of age grades in these societies is that in pastoral societies people have to be mobile. As the herds and herders have to move over great distances to find water and pastures, it is therefore a useful division of labour, over and above the sexual division of labour, to specify social function by age-linking dispersed herders into fighting groups for predation and defence. The relationship between different age sets also provides a generalized mode of behaviour that enables people to relate to each other socially when no immediate kinship ties can be found. Thus members of an age set are meant to respect members of older age sets as if they were their fathers or grandfathers, and receive respect from their juniors in a similar manner to that from their sons. Age grades help integrate the otherwise fragmentary kinship units, by creating cross-cutting ties that would help contain conflict between kinship groups. In tribal societies whose basic structure is formed through descent (particularly *unilineal* descent) and thus where people are divided into exclusive groups by affiliation through either the male or female line, groups define their social relationships to one another in terms of kinship. Ancestors become particularly significant and sacred because they stand for the social system. The genealogical relationships between the ancestors are thought to define the actual social relations in the society. Therefore the elders, who are those who are closest to the ancestors in the kinship system, share in their sacredness. They are not only the most spiritually powerful people, but can be the most influential politically, in that they have the longest memory of genealogical connections and can legitimize them. Furthermore, in a descent-based society they are likely to have the most descendants and therefore strategic political roles.

It is important to note that initiation into an age set is often accompanied by a painful ordeal, which is ritualized and marks the transition from childhood to adult status (La Fontaine 1985). However, this initiation is not compulsory when a person reaches a certain specific chronological age. Evans-Pritchard (for the Nuer) and other commentators rather point out that initiation is voluntary; the boy himself decides when he is ready to become a man and asks to be initiated (Evans-Pritchard 1940). Age-grade systems are not, therefore, strictly groups defined by members being of the same chronological age; although they are all of roughly a similar age, it is social age that matters. Further, it is the social chronology of age set succeeding age set that people use to conceptualize and understand their society and its history. Events are memorized by reference to the social events, the rituals, when particular age sets did certain things. One of the anthropological messages from comparing this kind of society to Western societies is how time, age and generation are socially constructed.

In some modern states, compulsory conscription for national service provides a not dissimilar function to age-set initiation. For the individual, it provides a ritualized transition from childhood to manhood; and for the society, it provides a method of promoting national unity by mixing people of different backgrounds in one universalistic (or at least nationalistic) institution with strong methods of socialization. The experience of military service is something that differentiates different cohorts in Britain and also provides contrasting experiences in different European and North American societies. Those who did national service in Britain or were drafted in the USA carried the mark of this experience through life. Some European states still have universal conscription in the late teens. Certainly many Bosnian elders were shocked to discover I had not done military service and had never carried a rifle. This they saw as undermining both my masculine and adult status.

Eisenstadt (1956) suggested two mechanisms by which age was likely to become a significant method of social solidarity. First he suggested that age groups tend to arise in those societies whose methods of social integration are mainly "universalistic". Although he is not simply presenting a traditional/modern dichotomy, this hypothesis is clearly an attempt to understand the developing youth phenomenon in post-war America by identifying youth movements as having a social integration function in transition from family to work. "Their function is to extend the solidarity of the kinship system to the whole social system through emphasis on diffuse age-group membership." (Eisenstadt 1956 quoted in O'Donnell 1985: 7)

Thus it is argued that age-group solidarity enables teenagers to move from the particularistic milieu of the family towards the universalistic world of work with the minimum social disruption. As a generalization across all societies this seems to have little strength in explaining the variety of uses to which age-based groups have been put. His second suggestion was that age groups tend to arise when the structure of the family, or the descent group, blocks the younger members' opportunities for attaining social status within the family. This seems a closer fit to the examples discussed in the next section on peasant households. However, these blocked status opportunities are a source of social conflict not of social cohesion. Neither of these ideas provide an adequate global empirical generalization or explain the development of the spectacular age-grade systems among the East African pastoralists. The East African age classes are not simple aggregations that facilitate social maturation; rather they form part of the formal institutional political and religious structure of society (Bernardi 1985: 148).

Peasant households

The third kind of society discussed in this chapter are peasant societies. In some of these societies ordinary elderly people also have the possibility of achieving relatively high status. Peasant societies are usually defined as being based on family labour in agriculture. One of the questions to be asked is: To what extent does the pattern of the extended family limit the use of age-related criteria in structuring people's lives? Are people perceived more on the basis of their familial position, as parents, children, grandparents, etc. in contrast to specifically age-based statuses? In peasant societies, extended families are quite common and there is a noticeable association between extended families and high status for elderly people.

I shall discuss the role of older people in rural Ireland during the last quarter of the nineteenth century and the first quarter of this century, as reported by Arensberg & Kimball (1940) and published in the *Irish Countryman*. In this society, which was characterized by high rates of out-migration, stem families became a common pattern. One explanation of this family pattern is that it was a strategy to keep small holdings intact in a situation where division of land through inheritance, threatened to reduce very small holdings to impossibly small holdings. There was a very late age of marriage and indeed high rates of celibacy. The son who was to inherit the farm could not marry until the "old man" was willing to retire, in which case a "match" could be made. This was a bargain, a legal arrangement, which would bring a wife to the farm along with a dowry. There was a circulation of dowry wealth, so that a family could afford a dowry for the daughter after having received one when the son married. The effect was a general raising of the age of marriage. In the agreement, the old couple retiring would specify the resources that they reserved for themselves from the holding, such as the use of a room in the house (the west room which Arensberg and Kimball suggest has mystical and supernatural associations); certain amounts of milk and vegetables from the garden might also be specified. When the old couple retired, a new couple could be married and take over responsibility but not before; so men in their forties were still "boys" because they were not married. Thus the key to status in this society was access to the limited amount of farmland and property. This meant that elderly people tried to control the farm as long as possible and it gave them authority over younger people in society and even over the middle aged. This society was not without its conflicts; the solidarity of the family, which was a prime social value, was riddled with the frustrations of the younger generations waiting for the old man to move on and give up the farm.

My own studies of such rural, agriculturally based societies have included not only rural west Ireland but also the alpine region of the Val d'Aosta (Vincent 1973a,b, 1987). In both these places familial institutions were as significant as the market and the formal institutions of the state in the organization of production. The village of St. Maurice had a population of around 500 people, who were distributed between a number of small hamlets varying in size from one to twelve families. At higher altitudes are the pastures, on which cattle are grazed in summer when the snows have melted. The commune depends largely on agriculture for its economy and St. Maurice, unlike other communities in Val d'Aosta, had enjoyed an expansion in its agricultural economy because of the building of a new irrigation canal in 1947–8 and the consequent enlargement of the area of irrigated meadow. Since 1960 there has been an increase in non-farm employment and the beginnings of a summer tourist industry. Transport facilities have improved; educational opportunities have developed; and consequently the commune has become more open to the influence of mainstream Italian culture and the European economy. The population is an ageing one, although permanent emigration has now virtually ceased and the young people are able to find economic opportunities, including farming, in the local area. In 1970, the commune was the site of a contested election between groups of candidates who were identified by the labels of "young" (*djuvieno*) and "old" (*viou*). This pattern of electoral contest has also on occasion taken place in other Valdotain rural communes.

The village society of St. Maurice was highly egalitarian between families. There was strong competition for status equality and not for status through ostentatious display. This equality may well have been the consequence of migration patterns, whereby the landless, without property ties to the village, left with the migration to America and rural-urban migration more generally. The upper classes either lost their status through the decline in the value of land or converted their status into education and the professions in which case they migrated to find career opportunities. This left as the core of the village the middle peasants, family farmers who held land and labour in some kind of balance within the family. Related to this competition for equality was the strong insistence on reciprocity. Favours were never proffered, only asked for. Thus there was always the expectation of reciprocity. Indeed, the reciprocity was elaborately institutionalized in many aspects of rural life. However, one consequence for elderly people of such values in this society was a tendency to social withdrawal. As has been the feature in depopulating rural areas in Europe, there was a high rate of celibacy in the village, and in addition there was no tradition of extended family living. Kin would live close, and married sons or daughters would even live within the same building, but as separate households. Even fathers and sons herding their cows together would know which animal was whose. Thus the very old, who were too frail to offer labour or other services in exchange, tended to withdraw rather than lose status. This was of great advantage to me as a visiting anthropologist because it meant that elderly people would be prepared to spend long periods discussing their life and their village to break the isolation and to establish a reciprocal relationship to which they could contribute. However, I had to work with the farming generation to persuade them to talk. Life-course events, including migration, and a relative decline in the rural economy, combined with a value system that highly values independence, left many old people lonely and isolated. This situation matches Dragadze's account of Georgian elders who, unable to maintain the requirements of the adult role which demanded responsibility for one's actions, tended to withdraw socially to avoid exposing their lack of socially expected control (Dragadze 1990).

The age-related features of the family farm economy in St. Maurice, namely the difference of interests between different family members and the ideology of harmony, came to the fore in the communal elections of 1970. The decisions that Mauricians had to make about development were both individual and communal. An innovation in local decision making was made with the administrative elections in 1970 to elect a Commune Council. This was the first contested election for the Commune Council since the advent of democratic procedures with the founding of the new Italian Republic in 1948. No previous election was contested, a panel of councillors being obtained by consensus. This 1970 election can be studied at a number of levels. It can be seen as a personality clash between the existing mayor and one of the councillors; a clash of interests between the "young" and the "old"; a conflict over the public reputation appropriate for a political leader in St. Maurice; or a move and counter-move in a political game in which the normative theme of *d'accor* (harmony) was used as a code for each attack and counter. It might also be seen as a clash between various neighbourhood and kinship groups. However, no single point of view reveals the whole picture. Local people can see subtleties in the ties of village and kin loyalty which would escape the most competent outside observer.

The two key concepts around which the election revolved were: how Mauricians see the ideal relationship among themselves, and how they view the relationship between their community and the rest of the world. The words by which these concepts are most frequently expressed in the local dialect are *d'accor* (harmony) and *en derrie* (backward). The rival factions each tried to justify their actions and their programme in terms of these key ideological features. The central issue in the election was that of development, particularly winter tourist development. Both sides acknowledged that the commune was backward. However, the "young" faction differed from the "old" in the remedies that it offered for this situation. These differences were seen locally in terms of personalities rather than policies. The electoral manoeuvring consisted of blackening the name of the other faction's candidates by spreading rumours. The talk in the bars was confined to laments about the failure to live up to the ideal of *d'accor*. However, these rumours reflected solutions to the state of backwardness associated with the different factions. The "young" were interested in winter sports, expanding job opportunities in tourism and good communications with Aosta. The "old" were more interested in the relationship with the regional government and the subsidies that might be forthcoming; they were concerned with roads for agriculture, for example a road up to the alpine pastures.

These rival definitions, both of the situation and remedies, reflect the generation gap and the differing life experiences of the young Mauricians from those of their parents. The major components of this different experience are educational achievement and contact with the world outside the commune. Of the twelve *viou* candidates, only two received more than an absolutely basic education by going beyond first or second grade. Both these candidates obtained an education via the only possible source at the time of their youth, through a seminary. These two candidates were the only ones on the *viou* list in non-traditional employment; the rest were farmers or craftsmen. However, amongst the twelve *djuvieno* candidates, all except three had received some training outside the commune. As a result of their education and training, only three of the *djuvieno* candidates worked as full-time farmers while all the others worked outside the commune every day – although the latter also worked on their families' farms. The older generation's view of tourist development was centred around grandiose projects financed from outside the commune such as the large winter ski station planned for the summer pasture. The *djuvieno* were directly interested in immediate, small-scale and more practical plans such as a small-scale ski-lift near the existing road. It is ironic that it was the more traditionally minded farmers in St. Maurice who should have been advocating the large winter sports complex as the route to winter tourist development. These farmers reasoned that the summer pastures were useless and covered in snow during winter. If used by tourists they would get some rent and perhaps a few other benefits, like roads, as well. They saw no costs to themselves in the project. The younger people, more familiar with the urban way of life, saw the irrelevance to their own needs of large complexes using outside capital, employing outside workers and used by short-stay foreigners. These young people could more readily conceive of risking their own money and effort in starting small-scale enterprises, catering for a localized market, in which they could work and from which they could reap a profit.

The *viou* won the election with a significant majority. One possible explanation for their victory was their stance on winter tourism.

They proposed a big development to combat the *en derrie* situation. This development was to be situated in a remote part of the commune, and so presented little threat to *d'accor* within the village. On the other hand, the *djuvieno* faction presented small-scale solutions, financed by individuals, which many residents saw as having less impact on backwardness and yet as also posing a threat to *d'accor* by strengthening economic individualism. In St. Maurice, although age grades were known and indeed, to some extent, institutionalized in an expected camaraderie among people of the same birth year, the political interest groups formed around age were the result of radically different cohort experiences.

Bosnian elders

I was involved in a study of the lifestyles of elderly people in Bosnia and Hercegovina immediately prior to the aggression of 1992. It was a society undergoing rapid social change. In the years after the Second World War it saw extremely rapid urbanization and industrialization; economic growth was accompanied by rural-urban migration and a decline in the subsistence peasant economy. One of the concomitant social changes was a move away from a family system, which was based around some of the largest extended household units found in Europe, to smaller family groups. Thus to some extent it is a case example of the impact of modernization on elderly people.

Despite the social expectations of the older generation, geographical and occupational mobility, as well as urban living accommodation predominantly in flats, means that it is difficult to sustain extended family living in an industrial society. However, this continuity is much more easily provided in the rural areas. Here, even if a joint household is not preserved, extended families live in different parts of the same house. It is also possible to build new houses on family land, so that the elderly have their children in adjacent property. Three kinds of family situation can be distinguished: one, in which the extended household is still intact; a second, where at least one child – usually a son and a daughter-in-law – lives either in a separate section of the same house or in a neighbouring house; and a third situation is found in those villages that have seen a massive out-migration (much of which has been abroad) and where only the old couple are left, with occasional visits from their children. It is in this last circumstance that the most difficult situations of social isolation for elderly people can occur. "The biggest problem for elderly people is loneliness. The elderly are used to having children around them and when they go they become lonely." (Bosnian social worker 1991)

The tradition of living in extended households in Bosnia can make elderly people feel lonely when they do not actually have people or children living with them in the same household. This can be the case even when they have many relatives living in close proximity or with children living in an adjacent house; elderly people can still feel that their expectations of joint living have been let down. Further, even within an extended family, elderly people can still experience grief at the loss of a spouse, kin, and friends or neighbours of the same generation. Many people can benefit from communal living, but it is wrong to over-idealize extended family living for elderly people. Extended families, like other forms of family, have their tensions and although daughters-in-law may do their duty, it is not necessarily the case that these relationships are without conflict.

Old people were vulnerable to poverty in Bosnia. Many people saw their lives as dominated by problems of survival in hard economic times. Respondents constructed their accounts by detailing "material" problems for old people, when they mentioned that elderly people have, as we would say in Britain, "difficulty making ends meet". Most people, identifying economic problems, would emphasize the low level of pensions and their unreliability. In 1991, because of the economic crisis in Bosnia, pensions had not been paid regularly for the previous six months and payments were falling further and further behind. One respondent said that "inflation meant that pensions and savings declined in value – unemployment affects the elderly through their children and grandchildren on whom they depend for support".

In the rural areas the problems for old people were not seen as different in essence from those of other people – all have to keep body and soul together. Families have to raise enough food, and live with the consequences of an overall low standard of living. Old people were subsumed in the family and not seen as a separate category. The economic problems for elderly people in town were seen to be rather different. They were thought to get better pensions, as many rural elderly were outside the enterprise-based pension structure. If urban retirees did obtain good pensions they were clearly substantially

better off than those living in the country, but there were concomitant problems of dependency. The pension ought to be reliable, paid
regularly and cushioned against inflation in a way in which it has not
proved to be the case in Bosnia. In 1991, at the time of the study,
Yugoslavia (and Bosnia perhaps even more so) was going through a
desperate economic crisis. Unemployment in some places reached 50
per cent; most people were on short-time or minimum wage rates,
inflation had been brought down from 3000% per annum to about
120%. The centrally planned economy located factories around each
locality in the republic for political and strategic reasons, which
meant that those towns that depended on one large socially owned
factory were particularly badly hit, as these enterprises were very
uncompetitive and there were no alternative sources of work. The
risk of outright starvation was avoided only because, in many cases,
the workers were also part-time farmers and could produce their
own food. However, the economic decline created great difficulties for
the pension system that is operated on a "pay as you go" basis and
was unable to pay existing pensions from declining salaries.

It is possible to summarize the relationship between urban industrial society and rural subsistence-agricultural society in terms of
their perceived consequences for elderly people. In the rural areas,
the use of the concept "age" was limited; there was no thought of
retirement and there was poverty. Those who were thinking in terms
of cultural continuity were working much more with the rural
community model, which did not differentiate age as a relevant
social category at all. However, there were those in Bosnia who identified a generational conflict, based on an urban conceptual framework of opposed interests of different sections of society for collective
goods and state resources, using the state as institution of redistribution. Those people who discussed the limitation of the social
infrastructure and the absence of old people's homes or adequate
mechanisms of social support; limited health facilities and access to
them; and basic infrastructure like roads and water supplies, were
thinking in terms of the industrial model of lifestyle for elderly people. Greater state provision was seen to be needed in the face of the
absence of family and communal resources that support people in
rural areas in later life. What this discussion of rural–urban contrast
in Bosnia tells us, is that life courses not only change between
cohorts – those who experienced migration to town were largely
the post-Second World War generations – but also that life courses

influence one another. The relative isolation or social support available to Bosnian elders depends on the life courses of their children and grandchildren and, in particular, their migration histories. The lifestyles of the different age groups are tied together in terms of economic redistributions between generations, even though the institutional mechanisms (such as pension schemes, or family gifts) may vary considerably.

The impact of modernization

How sources of social power and prestige for elderly people were undermined with the spread of capitalist society, is illustrated in all the societies discussed by their incorporation into labour markets and industrial economies. In all cases there was labour migration which undermined previous sources of status that were to some extent monopolized by the elderly in previous times. Fit young men left their societies to seek paid work: in the Australian Aboriginal case as cheap agricultural labour, on stock farms, ranching cattle and sheep; in the East African case, migration to towns, plantations, and to the mines occurred, as did commercialization of herding strategies. In Ireland there was a great outflow of labour to the growing industrial cities of America and Britain; from Val d'Aosta it was to France and the USA; in Bosnia it was to the towns or to the booming German economy. In the Australian outback the young men were able to gain wealth beyond the experience of their societies. The old men could not compete with such wealth, and outrageously juvenile men were able to attract women to live with them. The respect due from the young to the elderly was undermined and conflicts over women became more acute (Sansom 1978). These societies experienced radical social dislocation and anomie. French anthropologists discussing the impact of labour migration in West Africa on what they call the lineage mode of production point to the destruction of relationships between the generations. The power relationships and the patterns of social accumulation structured by kinship are dislocated when the young men are enticed away to wage labour for capitalist enterprises elsewhere (Meillassoux 1983). In the Irish case, access to land became less important as paid labour in industrial cities promised a better economic prospect. In many cases this meant that it was not the eldest son who had the option to remain on the land while his siblings were forced to migrate or remain unmarried, but the youngest son. The last son remaining, when the others had left to seek their fortune elsewhere, had to shoulder the responsibility of the farm and the old couple. The processes of modernization that undermined the social and economic significance of land and agriculture also undermined the social prestige of the senior generations in land-holding families across Europe.

In this chapter I have presented a view of the position of elderly people in a range of societies. Many of these societies might be labelled simple, traditional or even "primitive". These labels are unhelpful and stigmatizing. It is important to emphasize that I am not presenting the view that age is a respected status in simple societies and things go downhill in modern industrial societies. The situation is much more complex and the traditional/modern dichotomy confuses so many issues that it is not, on the whole, a useful set of concepts, certainly not when considering the elderly and their place in society. The next chapter, which concentrates on historical changes in the life course in societies with a European tradition, should not be read as presenting a model of how all societies will change. Furthermore, such a focus should not be taken to suggest that there are, on the one hand, unchanging traditional or primitive societies where the life course does not change and, on the other hand, modern societies with history and changing life-course trajectories to be studied. It is important not to make the ethnocentric mistake of seeing changes in the social position of elderly people from an entirely European perspective.

As a resident anthropologist in St. Maurice, age was one of the things over which I experienced culture shock and to which I had to adjust. In this small community there was a wider age range of people participating in a broad range of common activities than my British experience had led me to expect. My own experience of school and university was of very age-specific friendship and common activity. For example in sport, playing football was characteristically done with people of the same academic year as myself, or at most one year older or younger. This relates to the institutional practice of large groups of a common age forming a cohort progressing together through the educational system. However, playing football in St. Maurice the team was made up of people whose ages ranged from 14 to 30. What mattered was your familial position; whether you were a

young man not yet married, and had been to school in town; everyone, in that category joined in, even though some were twice the age
of others. The structures that produced narrow age cohorts in my
own society, particularly education, and rapidly changing popular
cultures, were not strongly present in this small-scale farming community. It is a feature of our late industrial society that kinship and
marriage are not nearly as important as in these other societies in
distributing the basic key productive resources by which a society
produces wealth. We live in a highly mobile society; most people own
no significant property. Although house ownership is growing, this
is not a productive asset that generates wealth but a form of consumption through which people find somewhere to live. Most people
have to find a paid job in order to survive and earn money to live.
Therefore embedded in modern capitalist society are pressures by
which elderly people without property and without work tend to
have little social status.

It is possible to conclude that there are sound material explanations for the social circumstances in which elderly people do not
become dependent on others. It seems, in particular, that where
capitalism creates a so-called "free market in labour", many of the
social processes that give status to elderly people are undermined and
elderly people are subject to exclusion from work that provides a key
to power and status. However, these explanations also need to
incorporate complex cultural and historical processes and simple
developmental models are inadequate. Most significantly, we can take
from this comparative study the view that comparisons of life
courses are a technique that can reveal the complexity of the relationships between differing groups in society and the status implications of these relationships. Life courses are structured both by
cultural meanings, applied to sequences and changes through life,
and by the material opportunities available to different sets of people.
The next step in this study must be to consider how the current
Western life course has developed.

CHAPTER THREE

Changing life-course patterns

As we will see in this chapter, the life-course approach developed in social gerontology is a highly effective tool not only in understanding the social situation of elderly people but also for the study of social processes in general. The idea of the life course, which includes that of cohort succession, facilitates the integration of a historical perspective into the debate on social inequality, without losing the individual perspective (Harris 1987). Thus, inequality as a feature of life courses will provide us with a powerful intellectual tool with which to reconceptualize processes of social inequality in general. The idea of life course is important because it enables us not only to look at elderly people in relationship to other age groups, but also in relationship to the historical development of the society of which they are part, and the place of their own personal biography within that history. Comparisons across time as well as across society will help reveal the processes that structure people's relationships according to age criteria. By reviewing changes in the history of the life course in Europe, and the Western world in general, we can start to understand the forces that lead to the current condition of elderly people (Van Tassel & Stearns 1986, Minios 1989).

The development of the Western life course

It is a common view that today's life course is more tightly scheduled and interlocked than in the past (Musgrove & Middleton 1981: 42), and that there is more regulation of life according to specific age norms (Hareven 1982: 15). Martin Kohli has used the term "chronologization" to describe the process by which the life course has become standardized across class, ethnic and gender boundaries (Kohli 1986: 271–303). Kohli suggests that chronology has come to have a strong grip on the life course of individuals. A process can be observed by which the criteria of age come to structure society, and relations within it, as a self re-enforcing process, and whereby the pattern is reproduced in stronger form over time. However, data presented in the previous chapter suggest that the life course in its current form is specific to the circumstances of modern, industrial, capitalist, society. The argument, therefore, is that in industrial society in the last part of the twentieth century, age is becoming much more important in relation to people's experience. It is becoming a criterion that more people use to interpret and understand their experience of society and to structure their own consciousness and action. It might also be suggested that it is not only age-based criteria through which the increased chronological structuration of contemporary life occurs, but that generation and cohort criteria have also become more socially salient.

Simplistic modernization accounts suggest a unilinear transition from tradition to modernity. Such accounts identify changes for elderly people as being from high status in pre-literate societies to low status in "advanced" ones; from ascribed roles in traditional societies to achieved roles in modern ones; from high status in agricultural societies to low status in urban ones (Cowgill & Holmes 1972: 323). Fortunately more sophisticated theories are available. Grillis (1987) rather suggests a three-phase pattern of change from an early modern period that he dates as 1600–1850, to a modern phase 1850–1950, which subsequently leads to the contemporary life cycle. He characterizes the early modern period as having an indifference to numerical age. The "ages of man" were socially not numerically defined and were conceptualized as being supernaturally, rather than naturally, determined. The evidence he adduces for this includes the variability in significance attributed to birthdays as events that mark an individual chronology. This contrasts with the celebration of "name days" (whereby those called John will celebrate the feast of St John, or a family will honour the day of their "family" saint), and patron saint days (whereby a community honours its special divine protector). Neither of these latter two ceremonies, unlike birthdays, are counted, they merely recur cyclically.

Grillis also found variability in the age of majority between classes and communities; there was flexibility in age of schooling – 14-year-olds went up to Oxford; and the age of military service and apprenticeship might vary. In this early modern period it was marriage that constituted adulthood and the age of marriage was normally later than is current in the late twentieth century. Marriage was regulated in families, not by age, but by birth order. Because age did not give automatic access to adulthood, he argues that a sense of life course as an orderly progression could not develop. He suggests that birth, apprenticeship and marriage were highly ritualized, because the rituals were required to create a sense of identity with the role; a sense of identity which age by itself could not secure. The notion of the steady development of a "career" was also discouraged by the character of the early modern economy, which did not assign tasks on the basis of numerical age, but on the grounds of status. Even in family matters, age was not a strictly determining factor. Frequent death meant that families were constantly reconstituted. Grillis says "step-parenting was frequent and parenting itself must be described as extensive rather than intensive undertaking . . ."(Grillis 1987: 101). The idea of childhood itself was blurred by the fact that it was a status – that of a minor – shared by offspring with the apprentices and servants of the household.

In the early modern period, Grillis goes on to suggest there were different notions of the self, which enabled people to step out of roles and assume role reversals, for example reversal of gender status in ritual form at carnival, etc. He sees the Puritans as changing this with their linear view of life, and their perception that such rituals were a violation of the true self. The stress in theology of the individual conscience, typical of Protestantism, required an individuated self. Cole (1992) elaborates a similar point of view, stressing how the idea of a vocation under Protestantism came to give meaning to old age, by viewing life as a spiritual journey culminating in a predestined triumphant end with salvation.

Historically the growth of individualism has been linked to the rise of the modern world. For Cole (1992), the growing interest in the individual is best understood in conjunction with the "spirit of capitalism", described by Max Weber, and the "civilizing process", described by Norbert Elias. The generalizing of the priestly vocation, discussed by Weber, which saw each individual life, from birth to death, as a sacred career, developed alongside new commercial ideas about time and work, together with specifically Protestant notions of salvation, and the gradual postmedieval shift of social context from the community to the individual. Arthur E. Imhof (1987) argues that the increasing certainty of living a full life span made it possible to think in life career terms, which in turn made people less imbued with *Gemeinschaft* values, because they saw themselves as individuals rather than as having a purpose as part of a larger whole. In other words, the rise of individualism had consequences for the later stages of the life course. Importantly, the condition of elderly people could then be seen as the consequence of moral choices they had made earlier in life. Victorian moralists proclaimed that morality determined the ageing process. Anyone who lived a life of hard work, faith and self-discipline would preserve health and independence into a ripe old age, followed by a quick painless natural death; only the shiftless, faithless and promiscuous were doomed to premature death or a miserable old age. However, the Calvinist self-confidence as the elected of God did not survive the secularization processes of the nineteenth century.

> By the late nineteenth century, the dominant culture of middleclass Protestantism had itself lost the ability to face ageing and death with existential integrity, bequeathing science a legacy of fear, evasion and hostility toward ageing. Indeed the core of this book shows how nineteenth-century Protestantism's growing commitment to Victorian morality and scientific progress undermined its ability to understand and accept the intractable vicissitudes of later life. (Cole 1992: xxv)

The "civilizing process" reached a high-water mark in the Victorian upper classes. In spite of severe social pressure for self-restraint, the ageing body posed intractable problems for the ideology of self-control. New methods in science and medicine appeared to offer, with their power and success in controlling untimely death, a secular rationale for how people should age. Cole (1992) argues that longevity and final chronic illness are consequences of modern scientific enterprise, but further states that the peculiar pathos of ageing in American culture derives from our denial of this new fact. Although it might be argued that it is more accurate to see medical science as probably of rather less consequence for longevity than economic prosperity, food production and sanitary engineering, Cole's key point about the shift from religion to medical science in determining the significance of age remains (cf. Kirk 1992); as does his recognition that medical science can never provide an answer to the moral and social significance of old age and death.

It is the work patterns of industrial society that are most frequently seen as setting the terms of the modern life course. Life courses in modern societies vary, but they vary within a basic framework. That basic framework is largely set by issues of material security; the stages of the life course are produced by definitions imposed by employment structures and the state. The development of a structured life course through the institutionalization of a retirement age is frequently dated in Britain to 1906 with the first pensions scheme, when support for retirement based on specific chronological age was introduced. It is the state that standardizes life events such as schooling and pension ages. The strong chronologization by the state in turn derives from the organization of production, in particular the divorce of the labour process from the family and the creation of a labour market, with the subsequent need for the state to intervene to set the conditions for stable control of the labour process. Hence it is suggested (Kohli 1990, 1991) that a powerful threefold chronology of pre-work, work, and post-work develops. Schooling and retirement are key transitions, largely set by the state, around which people's lives are organized. The transition from work to retirement in capitalist society is structured by the labour market, and is thus an inevitable transition that must occur, although the age of the transition is not necessarily fixed and can be related to contingent features such as an ageing society and the supply of labour.

The increased salience of chronological age in modern times is not simply true for the oldest generation, but also revealed in the way in which youth has developed distinctive lifestyles. There is a developed literature on youth culture, for example that produced by the Birmingham University Centre for Culture Studies (including Willis 1977, Hall & Jefferson 1976, Hebdige 1979). This work arose in response to specifically youth-based cultural phenomena. The development of the life stage now known as adolescence came with the development of modernity. In the nineteenth century, confirmation became part of church procedure, both Non-conformist and Anglican, emphasizing individual choice in faith, rather than the ritual of baptism, as entry into the Church. In these circumstances choice of faith had to await the life stage of an active moral conscience. Schooling became more regulated. The state started to administer school attendance and national conscription by chronological age. These changes can be seen as part of the bureaucratization and standardization that accompanied the rise of the nation state, but also linked to the growing emphasis on individual conscience. Moral responsibility required a period of guidance before full adult responsibilities and decisions could be taken. Consequently, a pre-adult life stage for those who were past puberty, but not yet fully adult, became elaborated.

The category "teenager" developed in the specific circumstances of post-war Anglo-American culture, and specific sub-cultural styles developed, associated with highly visible oppositional symbols and specific age groups. Willis (1977) and others argue that there is a class and family basis for the way in which teenage sub-cultures come to express themselves in opposition to adult and dominant class values. It remains an intriguing social question as to why older age groups did not also develop similar distinctive oppositional sub-cultural manifestations. If it can be argued that youth consciousness developed into forms of expressive cultural opposition to family authority and class oppression, can a parallel argument be developed, which refers to elderly people developing a pensioner or geriatric consciousness? Why did no emergent cultural opposition develop to the ascription of low status in old age? Was it that no real conflict of interest existed, or that the power of the dominant age group enabled it to secure cultural hegemony? Was cultural expression, in this case, so strongly determined, that no opposition could be manifest? The medicalization of old age has become so powerful during this modern period that it can be seen as a form of cultural domination; as a process structuring people's perceptions of old age and thus the possibility of creative cultural activity around old age. The differentiation of medical treatment for the elderly from treatment for other sections of the population is not simply a factor of the prevalence of disease, but of the cultural expectations of old age (Glaser & Strauss 1965, Henwood 1990). The study of the rise of Alzheimer's disease as a diagnostic category by Ann Robertson (1991) shows how, historically, institutional processes have elaborated the category "senile" in ways that structure and control elderly people. Are there no manifestations of symbolic opposition to such social determination by age or are we merely blind to them?

A key feature of the development of modern society has been the development of values associated with liberal democracy. Kohli (1991) argues that the use of age-specific rights runs against many of the universalistic tenets of liberal bourgeois ideology, for example that all individuals should be equal before the law. In practice, of course, some people are not equal because of their age. He cites struggles in America over compulsory retirement ages, which were seen as conflicting with anti-discriminatory legislation. The issues surrounding the Children Act in Britain, which granted children rights independent of, and potentially in conflict with, those of their parents, are a parallel example of the conflict between universal and age- (or generation-) based rights. Grillis (1987) draws attention to the differential gender and class implications of historical changes in the life course involving the individual, family and work. He suggests that females experienced a later chronologization of life course than men, related to the cultural priority given to earlier marriage, domesticity as opposed to employment, and regulation of female functions of reproduction. Although the female life course in the current era may now be seen as decomposing, with role switching between job, child rearing and parent care, in the last quarter of the twentieth century, divorce and remarriage make step-parenting more common, in parallel to the earlier model of the life course.

Prospects for the life course in the West

What are the prospects for the Western life course for the next century? Changes in families and changes in work patterns will have significant effects on the life course of succeeding cohorts. The increasing proportion of elderly people, and the increasing rate of family separation and recomposition, are trends found not only in Britain but also in America, Europe and the developed world in general (Johnson 1988a,b, Finch 1989, Goody 1990). How do these trends interact, and what will be their impact upon future life courses? There will clearly be different effects for different cohorts and different generations. Although it may be the middle generation, rather than those who are currently old, who are actually doing the divorcing, there will also be consequences for the younger generations, and further and different consequences for the oldest generations. These features, and particularly the last, are under-researched. What will be the impact of the recessions and unemployment experienced by younger cohorts today, when they reach retirement and old age? Pension companies, and governments keen to promote private pensions and savings, are systematically raising fears about the kind of pensions, health and welfare provision that will be available in the future. Clearly within current rules and welfare structures, which in Britain and elsewhere in Europe (Hugman 1994, Walker 1993) depend substantially on insurance contributions and a work record, high levels of unemployment and in particular youth unemployment will have lasting effects.

Migration patterns will also have severe consequences for future generations of elderly people. The rural-urban migration and the ageing of the countryside is a worldwide phenomenon (Sen 1994: 10). The increased distances of migration may be offset by cheaper and easier travel. Thus intercontinental migration may not limit generational interaction; because of expanding communications technology, and because jumbo jets and transcontinental motorways may facilitate on-going contact. However, the social barriers erected by cultural assimilation of long-distance migrants also disrupts intergenerational expectations. A rapidly growing proportion of the world's population are displaced persons – involuntary migrants. Such social dislocation will have consequences for the old age of those displaced, and further effects on those left behind. Periods of war and social upheaval also clearly affect the standardization of the life course. There is evidence that the cohorts who were starting their employment when they were disrupted by the Second World War carried the consequences of that disruption for the rest of their careers. Similarly, the marriage chances, and thus life-course patterns, of many women of marriageable age during the First World War were structured by the slaughter on the battlefield; life-course effects that are still felt today by that cohort. These consequences might be thought of as relatively minor perturbations in an overall system. However, what is claimed by the postmodernist perspective is that there is an overall de-stabilization of social structures and previous bases of social predictability.

Life-course patterns in the West over a 200-year period do appear to be more determined by age than in the past, but certain writers have started to suggest that this age-determined life course is now starting to break down. Elderly people are now able to choose from a wide diversity of lifestyles. Featherstone & Hepworth (1989), writing from a postmodernist perspective, suggest that the life course is becoming de-structured. Common social patterns determined by chronological age are becoming less critical to people's life experience. For example, there have been significant changes in retirement; early retirement has much expanded, depriving the age of 65 for men of its watershed character (Kohli et al. 1992). In the last two decades retirement age has dropped and Anne-Marie Guillemard (1989, 1990) suggests that, not only is the age of retirement declining but, there is a whole loosening of the life-course grid. Early retirement is more popular these days with firms, workers and the state, but as a response to the particular condition of the labour market and the growth in unemployment. Patterns of unemployment and early retirement interact, as do periods of unemployment, retraining and extended periods of education. If the age of retirement keeps coming down and the average age of leaving education keeps going up, somewhere about the age of 38 they should eventually meet. This proposition, which is of course impossible, serves to caution against simple extrapolation of current trends into the future.

Postmodern trends, which identify a de-structuring of the life course, suggest there is a reversal of chronologization. For example, marriage is becoming less of a key transition, as couples not only live together but many have children without marriage, and divorce and separation are increasingly frequent. With increasing longevity, fewer children and an increasing divorce rate, Bengston (1990), using California as an illustration of the future, has suggested that the new family is the "bean-pole" family. A family spread over four or more generations but with few members in each. This new family structure is clearly affected by such things as age of marriage, and age of childbirth, which are in turn strongly class related. The experiences of racial and ethnic minorities in America have produced family histories, and life-course expectations, at variance with the dominant Anglo-Saxon Protestant tradition. However, these patterns are also changing. In some groups, including Hispanic American and Chicanos, the age of childbirth has been coming down. Bengston notes that the mean age of the birth of the first child to Los Angeles mothers was 17, and also that the majority of women in the United

States who experience their 60th birthday this decade will still have a mother living. He thus foresees families of many generations, but relatively few members in each generation. As a consequence of such changes in family structure, the tensions of the nuclear family are now spread over longer periods of time and between fewer people. The implications of this are higher divorce rates, separations and perhaps more frequent pathological family experiences.

Postmodern work careers

It has been argued (Grillis 1987) that men were the first to resist chronologization and the impact of age-structured constraints. In schooling, the development of the mature student and repeated retraining blurs the association of youth and education. The occupation-structured male life cycle, it is suggested, becomes more flexible through more frequent job changes, forced and voluntary. Britain has seen a set of trends by which male life-time employment has declined, male self-employment has increased, and part-time work (particularly for women) has expanded considerably. The female life course may also now be seen as decomposing, with switches between job and work roles, child rearing, care for elders, and return to education as mature students. Although these trends are clearly evident, it may be that Grillis is somewhat romanticizing them, presenting them as choice and liberation, when they may merely be the consequence of economic failure, and the lack of alternative means to achieve cherished goals. Part-time work for most people is better than no work at all but not as good as permanent full-time employment. However, it can also be reasonably countered that there are considerable changes in the work ethic in contemporary society, and that such simplistic assumptions about the desirability of work need qualification.

Martin Kohli has been an intellectual heavyweight in developing a history and a prognosis of the Western life course. He poses the challenging question: Is an age-irrelevant society possible? The creation of such a society, in which no account is taken of age, would seem to be a form of Utopia in which ageism had been eliminated. For example, educational opportunities would be available to all irrespective of age. The transition from work to non-work would be voluntary, intermittent and not seen as retirement. What constraints exist on creating such a Utopia? Could we move to a situation where people could choose to retire when they liked; a position that would break the threefold pattern, of pre-work, work and post-work? Unfortunately this pattern does seem very resistant to change, perhaps because it is related to public pensions policies and the core of the compromise between capital, labour and the state, characteristic of modern industrial societies. It appears that up to the 1970s the institutionalization of retirement age at 65 (60 for women in Britain) was a clear pattern. Notwithstanding the last two decades, where the retirement age has dropped, what appears to be happening is that the threefold pattern remains but the dates of transitions are more flexible.

Kohli questions why partial retirement is not a more popular move in the life course. It is only in Sweden that this has been seriously tried. In America, mandatory retirement age has been abolished. However, this might have been easier in America than in the European welfare states, where comprehensive state retirement pensions are the norm, and that arose in response to the power and demands of organized labour. There are partial retirement schemes, for instance in Japan and Hungary, but the failure of this option more widely, suggests the threefold grid is still strong (Kohli et al. 1992, Johnson & Falkingham 1992). Given a capitalist society and the labour market which is inevitably a part of such a society, the transitions in and out of employment must occur. However, the age at which these occur is not necessarily fixed at any one point, and will be required to change according to demographic features such as an ageing society, and migration and the supply of labour.

Postmodern family careers?

What implications do the postmodern trends, which identify a de-structuring of social regularities, have on the patterns of family transition across the life course? The reversal of the pattern that Kohli has called "chronologization", may be identified in sequences of household formation and dissolution. Contemporary values place an emphasis on personal growth as a life-long process. Love is no longer necessarily seen as a once in a life-time event, something that occurs in late adolescence, the consequences of which have to be borne for the rest of one's life. Postmodern society offers a variety of individualized and love-orientated codes of values, in which people continually seek self-fulfilment and personal growth throughout life. These values can be seen to relate to changing patterns of family creation. Divorce and remarriage make step-parenting more common. The changing transitions in middle life are undergoing an increased ritualization process with 40th and 50th birthdays, or divorce absolute, or the anniversary of first meeting one's lover constructed as special ritual events marked with special ceremonial.

How does divorce/separation among their children affect the way that elderly people live? Some studies have examined how relationships survive, and how new ones are negotiated (Johnson et al. 1988, Finch & Mason 1990). What are the consequences for the older generation of such disruption, especially if it frustrates life-cycle expectations? It has been suggested that continued relations with in-laws by divorcees reflects four features: a long history of reciprocal support, and desire to facilitate contact between grandparents and grandchildren; good relationships while the marriage lasted; a divorce process that consolidated rather than undermined that relationship; and finding an acceptable basis for the relationship after the divorce (Finch & Mason 1990). There are clearly differential consequences for the social support networks of elderly people who have experienced these changing life-course patterns; they may be expanded with a new set of relatives or diminished by severance of valued ties. Some relationships can be sustained despite the rupture of links in the chain of affiliation. Johnson (1988a) has suggested that variation in the social and kin networks of divorced people affect their adaptation to family recomposition. New expectations and changes in broader social patterns are created by the spread of separation followed by household recomposition. To add to the scene of postmodern deconstruction, it has also been suggested that accompanying increased frequency of family recomposition there is a blurring of boundaries between generations and kinship roles, grandmothers may come to act as mothers, daughters like sisters (Johnson et al. 1988).

Studies that have looked at the role of grandparents have tended to take a social welfare perspective, looking in particular at the social support provided across the generations (Qureshi & Simons 1987). Thus studies that have concentrated on divorce and problems of child care, have looked at the support provided by grandparents to succeeding generations. Studies of supportive networks, and relationships between adult women and their mothers, have tended to look at support provided to the oldest generation, to discover the implications for community care and welfare support (Wenger 1984, Quershi & Walker 1989). Indeed many discussions about developments in family-based care have commented on, but not necessarily examined, the future availability of family carers. But the postmodern decomposition of the life course means that grandparents are no longer necessarily old. Indeed great-grandparents are more likely to fit the stereotype of frailty and dependence.

There has been the development of "new grandparenthood" whereby middle-aged people are able to elaborate the role of grandparent while they still have the resources drawn from employment, and can develop relationships with their grandchildren over many decades in a way that was unlikely in the past. The lifestyle of this new grandparent generation is postmodern in the sense that it is more fluid and less determined than previously. Lifestyle, in this context, is broadly conceived, not just as the term is sometimes used as merely patterns of consumption, but rather to indicate a complex of values and behaviour that is constructed by elderly people on the basis of their social location and the resources and life experiences they have available. The development of new roles and values, perhaps as step-grandparent or live-in great-grandmother, create opportunities for new lifestyles. Conversely restricted opportunities and resources, perhaps because of lost grandchildren through middle-generation divorce, constrain lifestyle possibilities. There are gender differences in lifestyles for grandmothers and grandfathers. Some studies have indicated that in addition to class variation in such roles, in some circumstances of family recomposition, grandmothers and grandfathers will substitute for the other role (Wilson 1987).

New and complex social situations are facing elderly people as the result of broad social changes in household composition and re-composition. These life-course changes will work themselves through in differing ways for different class, gender and cultural groups, and have varying effects on different succeeding cohorts (cf. Arber & Ginn 1991, Musgrove & Middleton 1981, Cribier 1989). While pension rights tend to remain with a male full-time worker and head of household, separated women are likely to experience a pension deficit in old age. In middle age, professional women may be spending significant portions of their salary to make up lost or limited pension

rights. Complex family structures mean complex inheritance relationships among the propertied classes, for example there will be
uncertainties about which of the grandchildren will have a stake in
the grandparents' property. These costs and incentives don't exist in
the same way for propertyless classes. Those with a cultural tradition
of the extended family may experience family separation and reconstitution as a greater trauma. Conversely, such traditions of family
solidarity may provide barriers to isolation and anomie for people as
they age. Cultural pluralism will be part of the experience of
postmodern society.

Deconstruction, disruption and cultural pluralism

Is it a mistake to look on family reconstitution as a feature of postmodernity? Can we compare family dislocation and recomposition
across cultures to gain a clearer idea of how it works and how it
affects elderly people? It is an error to accept too readily a postmodern perspective, which comes close to the moral right stance,
that society's values are breaking down, the loss of order is to be
deplored, and that the ephemeral has replaced the substantial. There
is nothing intrinsically traditional, or modern, or even postmodern,
about high divorce rates, step-parenthood or family dislocation.
Cultural changes and changes in values have to be located in social,
economic and demographic frameworks.

The dissolution of family units and kinship networks comes not
only from divorce but also from various forms of migration. Placing
these two trends in a comparative framework will enable the UK
experience to be located in a way that will assist in the analysis of
changing social patterns, particularly distinguishing cultural from
demographic factors, and cohort from generational effects on the life
course. How do people of different generations, genders, classes and
cultures construct the meaning of the disruption of their intimate
and familial social networks caused by recomposition of their children's households? How do the lives of those who are affected in parallel ways by widowhood or refugee status compare to "voluntary"
disruption of familial and household patterns by divorce or separation? What conceptualizations are made and what practical consequences result from network disruption by war and displacement as
opposed to divorce and personal motives?

Historically, some societies have had more fluid marriage arrangements than were found in Britain. Migrants from the English-speaking Caribbean have experienced significant cohort differences in family patterns. The reasons for these family patterns vary considerably and are the subject of debate. However, black families in the Caribbean, such as those studied by Edith Clarke (1957), Michael Horowitz (1967, 1971) and Nancy Foner (1976a,b), exhibit patterns of cohabitation, family recomposition, and late marriage. There is a wide variety of family patterns in the West Indies, characteristics of consensual unions, children born outside of marriage, and late age of marriage were common, along with an identified matrifocal family pattern with children brought up by grandmothers and maternal aunts. A wide variety of features affect these patterns. It has been suggested that the history of slavery destroyed stable family patterns, and in contrast that such patterns reflect pre-slavery matrilineal West African heritage. However, the most plausible explanation lies in access to land and secure jobs that could form a sound material base to marriage and these might only be found in later life. In those Caribbean communities where people had access to land and resources, marriage was the most dominant family form. Foner (1976b) suggests that with migration to Britain the tradition of grandmother care enabled both men and women to migrate in equal numbers in the 1950s and 1960s. In Britain the greater access to job and financial security meant that moves towards earlier marriage on the lines of the native society became more common. However, successive generations of West Indians suffered from being at the bottom of a society in economic crisis and women-centred families again became more common. This post-migration circumstance was frequently without the grandmother and kin support that was a feature of Caribbean social structure. Thus the interplay between migration and economic opportunity has meant that successive cohorts of West Indians have had different family life-course experiences.

Are matrifocal family patterns becoming more common among the majority populations of Britain, Europe and America to accompany the greater fluidity of household composition? This women-centred family pattern coincided with patterns of consensual cohabitation in many black populations in the Caribbean (Horowitz 1971). It remains to be established whether the growing patterns of consensual cohabitation and increased numbers of children born before marriage will lead to such matrifocal family careers. Some researchers have suggested similar features in the USA (Johnson et al.1988). Wilson (1987) writing about couples found no significant difference between maternal and paternal grandparental contribution to the support of their grandchildren. However, she suggests this may well be different for divorcees as opposed to the couples that she studied.

What happens in the situation of patriarchal extended families (which are the expected norm in many South Asian, Middle East and Balkan families) when divorce or migration disrupt the pattern of family succession? In this kind of family structure, the role of daughter-in-law is both potentially problematic and significant in the care of the senior generation. Even in Britain daughters-in-law are very likely to be carers for elderly people (Wenger 1984, Quershi & Walker 1989, Ungerson 1987). The family structures of South Asian families are traditionally extended and patriarchal, with early marriage for women and a strong antipathy to cohabitation. For example, the Punjab has a history of extended families, although here, too, considerable variation exists, not least between religious groups and between different classes. New families are not created on marriage, rather the bride moves into the groom's father's household and is usually under the direction of her mother-in-law in the performance of household duties. It appears more difficult for lower-class groups to maintain extended households, particularly where they are propertyless and dependent on insecure and inadequate wage levels. The mobile professional classes too may not maintain co-residence although very strong extended family loyalties remain that facilitate business links and migration. Punjabi migrants to Britain experienced considerable gender differences in the history of their migration. The extended families provided a haven for wives and children back in India. Thus men arrived first, and only subsequently were women brought over and families and communities re-established in the new country. Subsequently, new extended family patterns were established in Britain, sometimes involving bringing the grandparental generation from the Punjab (Sharma 1980, Khan 1976, Anwar 1979).

Here, again, the life-course experience of the different generations as the result of migration, family change and economic opportunity is significant; not only for interpersonal relationships within the family and community, but also in ways in which the communities interact with the host society and the welfare services in Britain. It is suggested that there are significant differences in the ways in which the senior generation of the West Indian community and the Asian community see the relationship between old age, ethnicity and the services they receive. The Asian community are more likely to see the need for specifically ethnic-related services whereas the Afro-Caribbean elders emphasize the need for services related to specific disabilities associated with old age (Blakemore & Boneham 1994, Askham et al. 1993). These attitudes are connected to the different language and religious needs of the Asian population relating to the historical difference in the two communities and how those historical traditions interplay with the life course. The South Asian extended families seem to be able to sustain familial relationships, including common budgets over considerable geographical distance. However, the effects of isolation caused by family dislocation can be very strong in people strongly socialized into collective family living.

The life-course approach to studying old age is particularly useful when looking at refugee elders. In these situations, it is necessary to have a framework in which to understand how the forcible disruption of expected life-course transitions comes to affect refugees in their later years. A brief examination of the situation of refugee elders from Poland and Bosnia currently in Britain will permit some comparisons. The Polish refugees experienced family dislocation early in the life course. As soldiers and exiles in the Second World War, unable or unwilling to return to post-war communist Poland, they saw dislocation during the period of early career and establishing families. The Bosnian elders currently being driven from their homes by ethnic cleansing also experienced conflicts during the Second World War and now have experienced even greater dislocation late in their life course. Thus, although both these groups of refugees may be of the same chronological age and at the same point in the career and family cycle, the impact of their forcible relocation will be significantly different. Many Polish refugees have remained unmarried or had restricted employment careers, or even remained in camps in the post-war decades. Their contemporary problems centre around returning memories of war-time events, and dilemmas as to whether to return to Poland after the fall of Communism. The Bosnian elders have been the most tenacious in refusing to move, because to do so is to abandon their life-time's achievement built into their homes. When they are forced out, the impact is one of despair and hopelessness. In old age there is little point in starting anew and adapting to the new location. The young refugees talk of moving to lands of new opportunity, using forcible migration as a labour migration opportunity. This is not available as a coping strategy to the older people. For the economic migrants who dream of retiring to their place of origin as prosperous pensioned successful people such a dream can have positive effects on adjustment to the low status and restricted opportunities of ethnic minorities. However, the Bosnian elders forced from their homes have neither economic opportunities nor the likelihood to "die in my own bed" (Vincent & Mudrovcic 1992, 1993).

This discussion of changing and alternative life-course experience required discussion of issues of gender, class, culture and ethnicity, as well as age. Conceptualizing them in the form of life courses has required a discussion of history. It is thus demonstrably a potent framework within which to make progress in understanding inequality.

CHAPTER FOUR

Old age and the symbolic order

In this chapter we examine the cultural construction of "old age". How are attitudes to old age embedded in language and the symbolic structure of Western culture? To place this discussion in context it may prove helpful to sketch my own cultural background, which involves moving from working-class London to English provincial academic life, as my own cultural repertoire and cultural interpretation will play a key part in presenting the symbolic structure of old age. There are two elements to the discussion. First the cues, the signs that are taken in social life to indicate roles and age-based categories. The second theme is the structure of the categories themselves. Thus the first part of the chapter attempts an empirical description, through observation and secondary sources, of how people are able to identify who is old. People "tell" who fits into the social category "old" in a similar fashion to the way they identify, using taken-for-granted assumptions, someone's ethnicity or class. The second objective in this chapter is to establish how "old age" is constructed in a pattern of meanings; how does the category "old" come to have meaning? Cole (1992) points out the dual meaning of "meaning", as cosmic significance–existential meaning on the one hand, as opposed to semantic meaning–the definitions of a term on the other. This chapter will reflect that division by conducting a semantic analysis, detailing a systematic pattern of contrasts, which map out the dimensions of the meaning of the term "old" (Black 1973, Vincent 1973b, Hymes 1964). By establishing that which the category "old" is different from, we can establish that which it is. The last part of the chapter is an attempt to assess the cultural meaning of old age in the cosmic sense; what intrinsic value, if any, is old age thought to have in our society?

Social cues to old age status

The social processes used in the creation of the social category of old age make use of law, appearance, behaviour, location, names and other cues. The life course in industrial society is pre-eminently structured by the state. The legal and bureaucratic mechanisms of the state allocate people into age-based categories. It is the transitions in age-based roles, recorded and legitimized by the state, which give the current life course its major stages, and make them concrete through bureaucratic procedures and certification. Claims made on the state for allocation of rights and duties have to be legitimated by appropriate documentary evidence of age. Access to school enrolment, driving licence, pension rights, exemption from jury service and a very large number of other aspects of social life require a birth certificate or evidence of a similar legal status of age. It becomes inconceivable, to those of us socialized in the bureaucratic West, that some people may not know how old they are. Many people in the world (but a rapidly decreasing proportion of people) were born when there was no mechanism for registration of births, so age could not be reliably established. Conversely in some circumstances, date of birth has become a key identifier for the state; in those communities and societies in which there are few alternative names in use and many individuals share the same name, date of birth becomes a necessary individuator. Bureaucratically organized signs can be used as symbols of old age outside the limited sphere of state activity and become cues for certain kinds of behaviour. Thus the pensioner is recognized by the pension book; producing a pension book not only entitles people to collect their pension, but acts as an access ticket to other resources as well, such as cheap prices at the cinema or in restaurants. The bus pass also stands as such a symbol; being ready to collect the bus pass shows a readiness to accept the age category "elderly", and is colloquially used by British elders to indicate an age transition.

Many of the cues used to categorize people into age groups are features of personal appearance. Visual markers that are taken to have some relationship to biological old age act as insignia. Grey hair is an obvious example. But sources of stigma can be reversed and turned into symbols of pride (Pratt 1976); as with the "black panthers", so the "grey panthers" extol as positive a usually negatively defined cue. Wrinkles, and the derogatory modern slang of "wrinkly", similarly links age and appearance. A stoop or an increased spinal curvature is frequently used when lay people are asked to role-play an old person. Various forms of visible or perceivable disability although not tightly linked to chronological age, still come to symbolize it. Thus problems with walking mean that a Zimmer frame or wheelchair become indicative of old age. "I am not ready for my wheelchair yet" may be used by people to reject their categorization as old. Failing hearing and sight can also be used stereotypically to indicate old age. Indeed failing health and fitness more generally, is used in self-definitions of age status (Thompson et al. 1990, Vincent & Mudrovcic 1993). Objects that are associated with such disabilities, hearing aids, walking sticks and the like, then become symbolic of old age. The European standard street sign that indicates "elderly people crossing" features a walking stick and spinal curvature. Mental states are also used as cues to old age and, in particular, failing memory is used to identify the social category "old". However, although depression shows an epidemiological pattern in which it is more frequently manifest in the elderly, this pattern of morbidity is not used in the same symbolic way as are memory lapses.

Because of the cohort effect, whereby certain styles and fashions become associated with particular age groups, some cues can derive from changes in fashions and can thus indicate old age. For example, first names tend to go in fashions and therefore old people can often be identified as such from their names. In Britain, it is reasonable to anticipate that people named Albert, Agnes, Doris or Fred are likely to be senior in years to those called Wayne, Sharon, James or Charlotte. Similarly, adherence to certain styles of dress, so-called "old-fashioned" styles, can indicate age cohort (Fennell et al. 1988: 11). Use and style of hats for example is often distinctive. Will being a card-carrying member of the Mick Jagger fan club have become a similar signifier of old age in thirty years' time? Recreational preferences, sometimes elaborated by commercial and consumer considerations, can also come to be expressive of the senior generation. Saga holidays, whist drives, lavender perfumes and many other behaviours come to have associations that connote old age.

Cohort effects and age stratification processes can mean that certain places and activities become associated with older people. As cities have developed, people have moved into new housing areas together. Frequently this move was as young people who then grew old together; so that certain former suburbs, now often in "inner city locations", are associated with elderly people. Some kinds of housing are constructed and allocated to specific age groups; housing for the elderly retired or sheltered housing. Similarly, some retirement locations like Hove, or Sidmouth, Harrogate or Tunbridge Wells become symbolically attached to old age; with such an address then comes a certain presumption of age (Karn 1977, Warnes 1982).

Cognitive categories and the structural meaning of "old"

One method through which to understand the meaning of old age is to examine spread and limits of the category old. By analogy with a map, a semantic space is the area covered by an idea; to know the content of the idea is to be able to define the boundaries of the semantic space (Goodenough 1964, 1968; Hymes 1964; Frake 1962). What are the contrasts between the concept in question and others? What are the essential characteristics that distinguish the meaning of the concept under discussion from other ideas? No term has meaning on its own; it is only when it is placed in a structure of meaning that it can make sense (Lévi-Strauss 1963, Douglas 1973).

What does "old" contrast with? What is the opposite of "old age"? It contrasts with both "young" and with "new". Hence "old people" can be thought of as the opposite of both "young people" and "new people"; the former meaning, for example, an age class or those below the average age of current audience, while the latter might denote people who have just moved into the neighbourhood or recently taken up a government position. Hence also, both "young age" and "new age" contrast with "old age" and illustrate the difference between personal or age-grade time, and historical or cohort time. A "new age" can mean a new historical epoch; it is possible, but unlikely, that a "young age" could be used in a similar fashion, it is much more likely to refer to a person or people (or possibly other living things).

Consider the following list of contrasts and examine what they indicate to us about the range of meaning of the category "old" when contrasted with "new":

- old days; good old days; times passed/new day; new dawn; modern times

  "Old days" are usually "the good old days", in contrast to the decline or decadence of the present. In this context, age is associated with tradition and positive values. "Modern", most frequently, has the positive meaning of progress, but not always – Charlie Chaplin's *Modern times* was a dystopia.

- old times sake; old love/new love; passed love

  "Old" applied in these contexts is a term that carries feelings of nostalgia, commitment and community. Because of the supreme value attached to the concept of love in the West, it is not easy to find words that carry meanings about its passing. Thus "old" in these cases does not carry a negative connotation.

- old familiar places; old familiar faces/new faces; new places
- old habits; old traditions; old ideas/new fashions; new ways; new ideas

  Age can venerate and sanctify traditions, values and behaviour, but it can also render them obsolete, outmoded and obstacles to progress and betterment. The "old country" is the place of origin, indicating also respect. Whereas the "new country" is the place of migration, which, if it is also a "young country", might be recently settled or recently independent. "New" not "young" is used for cars, houses, and even "new men" to describe a new regime or administration. "New women, new men" in the plural is suggestive of social change; in the singular "new man, new woman" of a person revitalized by sleep, a trip to the hairdresser or a religious experience. Although these patterns of meaning may suggest a positive side to "old", consider also the following:

- old-fashioned/in fashion; new fashions

  Here there are connotations of lack of progress, obsolescence; although reference to tradition and time-honoured values might also be being made. "You can't teach an old dog new tricks" – the old are seen as conservative in their ways, not flexible like the young.

- old shoes; old clothes/new shoes; new clothes; new lease of life
  old stale clothes/fresh clothes; clean clothes

  "Old" can have connotations of comfort and wear but also shabbiness and dirt. In this contrast it is opposed to fresh, clean

and polished; and by extension into a social analogy, with taking up existing or newly established roles or social position; a new broom sweeping clean the old regime. Also consider:
- old-fashioned clothes/young clothes
- old time dancing; old time music hall/new wave; modern dance; contemporary dance.
- old jokes/fresh jokes

These uses of the term carry the meanings of tradition and progress and sequences of fashion, that social and cultural knowledge is bound by cohort and "generation". "Old hat" has a particular meaning denoting a cliché, information passed its sell-by date. Old jokes are almost certainly bad jokes, lacking the element of surprise, but on the positive side having a tried and tested character to them. Thus the contrast "old" as opposed to "new" contrasts tradition and community with shallow fashionable modernity, but also indicates backwardness and obsolescence and contrasts with progress and originality.

The contrast of "old" with "young" produces a slightly different set of meanings and connotations. This can be illustrated when the terms are associated with the symbolic meaning of parts of the body. Consider the contrast:
- Young blood/old bones

This has meanings that imply reinvigoration, vitality and strength, as opposed to weakness and powerlessness. Whereas "young at heart" indicates the ability to retain the features of youth in later life.
- Young blood/old head

This contrast indicates the impetuosity of youth as opposed to the cautious wisdom of age. "Young" or "youth" has the connotation of immature, "wet behind the ears"; but age can harden and toughen natural things. "Old man of the sea" or the "old man of the mountains" implies close to nature, wild, tough, enduring; as opposed to "young man about town", the soft, sophisticated, cultured, fashionable.

What happens when the term "old" is applied to particular types and classes of people? There are some strong gender differences in the terminology. You can use "young" as in: young man, young woman, young boy, young girl, young person; but "youth" is usually simply male when used as a personal noun. What is associated with old man/old woman, as opposed to old person/old people? An old man can be a "dirty old man", with a sexual meaning; "dirty old woman" is a term less likely to be heard and is less likely to refer to sex. "Old dear" or "old biddy" is patronizing and carries female connotations; it is unlikely that a man would be referred to in such a way. Terms of abuse to women, such as "witch" or "old cow", although containing associations with age, can be used to women of almost any age. Similarly, animal images oppose young and old animals; kid, to old goat, or nanny. This has a sexual side, as with: young buck/old dog or old goat (note these are male words). "Mutton dressed as lamb" reflects both gender and ageist stereotyping.

Once people are sorted by cues which classify people, these people can be labelled.There are synonyms for "old" that have relatively positive meanings, and by analogy provide positive images of old people. These synonyms include:

- ancient, as in "ancient monument"
- vintage, as in "vintage wine" or "vintage car"
- antique, as in "antique furniture"
- veteran, as in "veteran cars", "veteran soldiers" and "veteran footballers"
- mature, as in "mature cheese" or perhaps a "mature artistic performance".

Hence, the "ancients" as a social group carry the meaning of ancient wisdom or valued ancestors. A "good vintage" might be used to refer to someone who has been thought to age well. Antique may also have meanings of fragile as well as old but is definitely valuable and so definitely more socially acceptable than old-fashioned. Veteran is definitely a positive term indicating experience and survival capabilities; old soldiers never die they just fade away. While an old car may be thought to be cheap and unreliable; a veteran car is expensive, collectable and likely to be well looked after. For an artist, a mature performance reflects the wisdom that comes with age.

Old age is so socially devalued that it is sometimes easier to avoid using the word altogether. Hence a variety of euphemisms develop which stand for old age, but attempt to take the sting out of the word. How do they achieve this? Consider the following euphemisms for old age:

- senior citizens: seniors have status and citizens' rights
- twilight years: twilight is romantic and avoids the black night of death
- elder people: elders have an association with seniority as in the

Church, elders are the respected leaders of the church in a former age
- Darby and Joan: these are model characters with whom one should be pleased to be associated
- Old dears: this is a term of endearment, generalized to the point of being patronizing

There are very many words which denote people of young age – child, baby, toddler, teenager, kids, bairns, brats, urchins, boys, girls, lads, lassies, maids, sprogs, etc. There are many (but less) terms for the older years. The use of kin terms, granny, gran, nanny, nan, pop, grandad, old man (meaning father or husband), is quite frequent. There are some "stage of life" words such as pensioner, senior citizen, old stager or veteran; and there are also some pejorative labels such as the modern "wrinkly" or the archaic "dotard". People can be referred to by decades; as in their twenties, or forties, or nineties. However, there is an almost total paucity of words to describe middle age or the prime of life. "Old" and "young" tend to be seen as the extremes; the beginning or end of the cycle. In other words, it is the middle that is seen as "normal" or the reference point. By implication it is the middle, the middle aged who are doing the defining. "Menopausal" or "mid-life crisis" are the only pejorative terms specifically associated with middle age and they also have gender undertones, that complicate their significance as indicators of age stereotypes. Language use seems to suggest a social dominance by the middle aged.

Many images of ageing identify life as a journey. This journey may be circular to a homecoming, or linear from disorder to order (i.e. salvation, redemption). The seven ages of man, which for example appear in Shakespeare, were widely used in early modern Europe, and image a cyclic progression from childhood to renewed childhood. When this is represented as a picture, the middle ages are shown at the top. The ages of life were also used as an image to structure medical concepts; certain humors dominating in certain ages. However, the dominant images of old age and ageing are images drawn from the natural world. These natural images include natural cycles and natural objects. Natural cycles have "young" and "old" phases. The moon waxes to a full moon but as it ages the old moon wanes until it is replaced by the new moon. The tides flood in and the neap or spring tide is at its height, but it ebbs and loses its force; a dying person is said to be "ebbing away". The diurnal rhythm dawn, day, evening, night is used to parallel age changes. Old age being seen as evening and approaching night as death. The riddle of the sphinx asks: what goes on four legs in the morning, two legs at midday and three legs in the afternoon? The answer is man, but the image is of ageing as the daily cycle from dawn to dusk. The seasonal round pictures old age as autumn and associates winter with death.

Many of the natural objects symbolizing old age then draw on this cycle for meaning, the tree and falling leaves denoting the autumn of life.

What more is man than the trees of the field?
A man has his seasons so why should he grieve,
    like the leaves we will wither and soon fade away. (Traditional)

The natural process of ripening, maturity and decay are also used to image old age; either as maturity or as decay. The terminology of age is strongly embedded in analogies with food: raw, fresh / ripe, mature / decayed, rotten, stale, gone off. Thus, old bread is stale as opposed to fresh bread; young wine needs to mature, and old –in the sense of vintage – wine is valued, but old wine that has gone stale or has refermented is no longer of any value as wine. Furthermore, in addition to biblical analogy – for example "old as Methuselah" (the oldest man in the Bible who could not die until he met with the Messiah) – extreme age can be indicated by the long-term natural processes of geological time ("old as the hills") or of biological growth ("long in the tooth").

The inanimate sense of "old" tends to mean worn or worn out, not working well, lacking in power. The mechanical analogy of the old, i.e. worn-out clothes or cars, contrasts with the organic analogy of the ripened fruit decaying with age. Worn or worn out is the association for inanimate objects that can be contrasted with natural cycles for animate things that rather decay. There are the images of old age that associate it with lack of vigour and force. This tends to be seen as a mechanical or impersonal force as opposed to organic or animate ones; the sands of time running out, the winding-down of the clock work. Rivers are imaged as young and vigorous in the mountains and slow and meandering as they get old near the coast. Similarly, the fire is seen to flicker into life, and become fierce flame, but dies away as it ages into embers. The analysis of folk concepts of ageing reveals that the structure of these concepts parallels the theories discussed in Chapter 2 on biological ageing. Two kinds of theory were identified: one sees ageing as "wear and tear", the cumulative effect of continuous use; and the life-span view, or biological alarm clock that rings at the end of the allotted time.

Structural analysis of age concepts

Both ageing and death also have a relationship to the social conception of time. Time is a socially organized and understood phenomenon. The experience of time slowing down when one is on holiday in a rural setting is an illustration of this fact. Two basic alternative concepts of time are prevalent; the arrow of time and the round of time. This is to say, some societies do not see the future as radically different from the present. Our society in the West is built around ideas of progress, and time is the history of that progress. The future, the time to come, is new and modern. Alternatively, some societies see various cycles, which revolve and recreate the same world, time and time again (Bailey 1971).

In the Australian Aboriginal world there are two kinds of time. There is sacred time; "dream time". "Dream time" was/is the time of myths and heroes, when sacred ancestors and creators acted/act out the key dramas of the universe. The other time is our time which is merely a shadow of these events. Our time does not change or progress but merely reflects what happened/happens in dream time. Individuals live a life that reflects that of their sacred ancestor precursors. People most in touch with the ancestors, who know most about dream time, through, for example, visions or being able to recite myths, are as a result somewhat special. Such people tend to be older (Berndt & Berndt 1983, Sharp 1952).

The Hindu vision of time is of cycles, wheels within wheels, *kharma*. The cycles of the universe are the *yuga*; our current Kali yuga being an evil time awaiting destruction and rebirth. The idea of an *atavar*, the current reincarnation in a cycle of rebirth, suggests death is but an interlude not an end or a final goal. The (male) individual should proceed through the stages of life from student, to householder, to aesthetic (*sanyassi*), to hermit. This ideal life course may not always be achieved, especially by the poor and the powerless in lower castes. However, such a sequence is required of those who wish, through self-knowledge, to break free from the endless cycles of time to reach a timeless release (De Bary et al. 1958).

Both these views of time contrast with the "modern" understanding of time. However, they differ from each other in the importance they place on sequence or marking or counting of time. Our modern Western society not only sees time as an arrow and (to mix the metaphor) marching forward, but something that is precious, must be counted and that must be saved. Watches, which can count in tenths of seconds or less are commonplace items of personal apparel. One logical consequence of this progressive view of time is that the significance of events is seen to fade as they pass into history; the longer ago something happened, the more it loses its significance. If time is not seen as progressive and moving forward, all of the past has a similar status; it is not differentiated. There is a story that when the colonial administration and police force were established in the southern Sudan among the Nuer, a man walked into the police station to report a murder and asked for the arrest of the culprit. The police officer was shocked to find that the event had happened thirty years previously. To the Nuer this time gap was irrelevant; to the policeman it radically altered his perception of the event.

Ideas of time clearly affect the understanding of the sequence of the life course. One might hypothesize that the close approach of oblivion and irrelevance would lower the status of elderly people. By the same token, where death is seen as translation into a more powerful or desirable state, higher status might be anticipated. How do cultural understandings about the nature of time affect images of ageing? It is possible to construct a fourfold classification of images of ageing (see Table 4.1). The two dimensions of the classification are, on the one hand, progressive (linear) as opposed to non-linear images of time (the arrow of time as opposed to the round of time), and on

Table 4.1 Classification of images of the life course and old age.

	Death and life as interludes	Death as the end
Continuous time not important measure	Continuity of all life courses (Aboriginal dream time)	A single life in ritual stages (European medieval view)
Sequential time is counted	Spiral existence of many life cycles (Hindu *atavar*)	A single life in stages by chronological age (Modern Western view)

the other continuous images (life as an interlude in the great scheme of things) as opposed to sequential images of the life course (the ages of "man").

This classification reveals the relationship between the conceptualization of ageing and old age, with the conceptualization of time and of death. The view that we only have one life and that this is marked by death at the end contrasts with the view of death and life merely being opposite sides of a cycle, whereby souls, or *atavar* have continuing existence. This is not a material versus a spiritual conception, because the single life ending in heaven or perhaps hell is a common conceptualization, indeed the dominant occidental one. While the significance of marking time or measuring the years to count age, as opposed to a view of age not as years or stage, but like a procession, is clearly related to the processes of chronologization discussed in the previous chapter.

It might be argued that the contemporary movement to have ageism opposed, along with racial or gender chauvinism, is an attempt to move from the lower to the higher section of the diagram. The effect of this is to limit the significance of chronological time, and thus age, in determining life-chances, and reflects a social movement away from highly regulated stages of life, to the "postmodern" attitude that everything is allowed. A genuine defeat of ageism would involve having choices about what age you wish to be!

Death and the meaning of old age

The idea of old age is intimately associated with the idea of death. *One foot in the grave* and *Waiting for God* are television programmes that are focused around age as an issue. Across different societies, the status of elderly people is closely tied to the status of the supernatural, and ideas of life after death. Thus understanding social attitudes to death and dying is crucial to understanding the meaning of old age. The cultural treatment of age is related to the cultural construction of death. However, death may be seen as passing from the cultural to the natural, as with the decay of the corpse, or as elevation to the supernatural as an angel, ancestor, soul, etc. These last concepts are, of course, archetypically cultural constructions and vary significantly from society to society. It has been argued that marginal characters, people or things that confound society's taken-for-granted categories, take on the character of being highly sacred or highly profane (Durkheim & Mauss 1963). Those between the world of the living and the world of the dead carry that ambiguity. If seen as profane, they may be rapidly disposed of by low-status, outcaste groups; or, if seen as sacred, they may be very carefully preserved and placed in a sacred site for public veneration (as was Lenin). Those who are socially nearly dead also carry the mark of their ambiguous position between the natural and the supernatural.

The contrasts that are believed to differentiate the natural from the supernatural are not the same, and indeed are very different between societies; it may be argued that some societies do not have the category supernatural at all. However, if the transition associated with death is conceptualized as being a return to nature, to a non-social condition, then the structural logic necessitates the creation of a devalued status for those in, or close to, that condition; dead bodies frequently arouse the emotion disgust in modern Western societies (Sudnow 1967). However, the dead, and even dead bodies, can also be revered when the transition is conceptualized as becoming supernatural, in a positive and sacred sense. Funeral rites can frequently be seen as an attempt to resocialize the dead, reintegrate them into culture (Bloch 1971, 1989). An extreme form of this is endo-cannibalism, where part of the deceased person's body is eaten by the living generation to preserve the material or spiritual essence of the dead person within the living (Donner 1982). The socialization of natural products into food is the subject of Lévi-Strauss's structural analysis *The raw and the cooked* (Lévi-Strauss 1970); the resocialization of the natural product of death – the cadaver – similarly requires a cultural apparatus. The argument here is that there is a universal pattern of association that links elderly people with death. However, the evaluation of these categories can be either positive or negative.

Psychological theories of ageing have tended to be more concerned with death and the immanence of death, while sociological theories have only recently touched on the issue (Elias 1985, Bauman 1992). There are some interesting studies that discuss the social construction of death, including for example Sudnow's (1967) work *Passing on* and Glaser & Strauss's *The awareness of dying* (1965). Death is more and more removed to specialist institutions such as hospitals and nursing homes. These studies show how death in these places is routinized and brought under the social control of professional specialists, such as undertakers. Numbers of sociologists have noted that the trends in modern society to rationalization, secularization, routinization and bureaucratization apply as much to death as to life (Clark 1993, Dickenson & Johnson 1993: i). Community skills in dealing with death have been lost; very few people in Western society would have any idea how to deal with a body of a dead person, and "laying out" would be regarded by most people with extraordinary repugnance. Death among younger people has become much less frequent, with the consequence that the elderly are the group in society among whom death is most powerfully associated, and people no longer experience death as a commonplace event, possible at any age. The secularization of society, and the youth-orientated nature of our culture, deprives death of social value, and people do not have the social resources with which to understand, and come to terms with, death in a routine or positive way. It might be argued that it is secularization in conjunction with this association with death that has led to the low status of elderly people. There is some force to the point of view that in contemporary Western society, our particular set of cultural values relegate the very old to the undesirable status of living dead. However, the idea that death, or association with the supernatural, is a bad thing is not from an anthropological point of view universally the case.

Therefore, a key problem for those who wish to attach more positive meaning to old age in contemporary society is the close association of old age with the devalued status of death (Mellor 1993). The inability of our society to come to terms with death has been discussed by a number of key sociologists including Bauman (1992) and Elias (1985). In *The loneliness of dying* Elias (1985) argues in a way that initially appears similar to functionalist disengagement theories (discussed in Ch. 8), but is based on a sounder understanding of social process, particularly historically located social processes. His approach to long-range social change lies in the idea of interconnectedness, long chains of social relationships that affect (but do not determine) each other. One such long-term historical social process he sees as the civilizing process, and he documents how social restraint of bodily functions and emotions have become more powerful and internalized. Fighting, fornicating, eating, urinating and the like have become more and more restrained by internalised social conventions (Elias 1982). These processes affect elderly people, and in particular the dying, where the internalized social control becomes less effective. People who cannot perform the required internalized control of physical functions and cannot exhibit the socially necessary restraint appear unattractive, dirty and undesirable; as if they were uncivilized. Further, social interconnectedness breaks down, and the anticipation of death alters the structure and consequences of elderly people's interaction. Elias identifies a historical relationship between contemporary social restraint – the politeness, the civility, of interpersonal exchange – and the strategic manipulation of self in courtly society ("courtesy"). In other words, manners are a way of managing a continuing relationship. The social strategy of civility is less effective if the relationship has no possible lengthy duration, and thus constructing new relationships becomes more difficult; and in the nature of demography, existing relationships will for the older person be increasingly terminated by death. By a similar logic of social strategy, the emotional investment in the relationships of elderly people becomes limited. No rational person would logically make their future happiness and emotional wellbeing dependent on someone who is not expected to live long. Hence the loneliness of dying.

Bauman (1992) suggests that contemporary society tries to deploy simultaneously two types of strategies to undermine the significance of death. The modern type has a characteristic drive to "deconstruct" mortality, by dissolving the issue of the struggle against death into an ever-growing, and never to be completed, set of battles against particular diseases and other threats to life. It thus seeks to move death from its previous position as the ultimate, yet remote, horizon of life span, right into the centre of daily life, as an ordinary technical problem to be coped with by known routines. Thus the defence against death becomes to change it into non-ultimate, relatively smaller, and thus in principle "soluble", problems of hazards to health. Counterpoised to this view is the postmodern, with its effort to "deconstruct immortality". This strategy involves substituting "notoriety for historical memory, and disappearance for final – irreversible – death, and to transform life into an unstoppable, daily rehearsal of universal mortality of things and of the effacement of opposition between the transient and the durable" (Bauman 1992: 10). These positions are of course contradictory, but are nevertheless employed simultaneously, not least in spectacular surgery, for example, where artificial hearts or new internal organ transplants are placed in patients with little chance of survival, but conducted in a blaze of publicity and media spectacle.

The value of old age

Thomas R. Cole in *The journey of life* (1992) typifies three ways of ageing based around differing ideals. These are:

1. the transcendence ideal in which the goal of ageing is to bring oneself into alignment with an order of the cosmos;
2. ideals of morality which articulate social behaviour considered necessary for a good old age and its religious rewards;
3. ideals of "normal" ageing that seek to maximize individual health and physiological functioning in old age through scientific research and medical management.

These three modes of ageing may be summarized as cosmic, social and individual ageing, and may be thought of as a historical sequence. In a powerful critique, Cole (1992) demonstrates the inadequacy of the current "individual" mode of ageing. He sees professional medical and welfare groups usurping people's ability to define their own problems, turning them into technical matters and thus depriving them of moral or spiritual significance. The dominance of scientific and technical knowledge (Habermas 1971) may enable us to prolong life but it fails to give meaning to the prolonged existence of ageing and, in some cases, dysfunctional bodies. Cole uses examples from his own family to illustrate the problem and to point up the relationship between public issues and private problems (Mills 1970).

> My grandmothers both felt a deep sense of shame and revulsion at their own failing bodies. These feelings reflect our culture's intractable hostility to physical decline and mental decay, imposed with particular vengeance on older women – which encouraged them to think of growing old not as a part of the human condition but as a solvable problem. (Cole 1992: xxiv)

Because all societies establish systems of meaning that help people orient themselves towards the intractable limits of human existence, to understand the meaning of old age it is necessary to understand the culture in which it is located, and how that culture has developed. If the problem of old age in modern Western society is the loss of meaningful roles for elderly people, then how is this loss of cultural meaning to be overcome? Growing old cannot be understood apart from its subjective experience, mediated by social conditions and cultural significance (Meyer 1988). What aspects of modern culture are amenable to reassessment in ways that can help redress the evaluation of old age?

The negative stereotyping of old age is called ageism. Stereotyping is simplified over-generalization accompanied by a rigidity of thought that imprisons others in a role. The negative aspects of that role have been the subject of this chapter. The opposite of ageism might be conceived of that which Germaine Greer (1993) has called "youthism", which is the "worship of all things youthful", i.e. a positive stereotype of the desirable attributes of youth. This obsession of youth in the culture of the contemporary West, she argues, deprives old age of positive meaning and identifies it as an undesirable state (Hilton 1993). Until people positively welcome reaching old age and do not regret the loss of youth, the low status of elderly roles will continue. This observation may have force, but the explanation of the origin of "youthism" is journalistic and ahistorical. In parallel to a number of ideologists from the right, she blames the 1960s generation and suggests it was the rebelliousness of that generation which rejected the values and authority of tradition. This, she argues, meant that the newness of youth became valued for its own sake; with the concomitant rejection of old age. The twentieth century has been a revolutionary century; in many places across the world there have been attempts to throw out the old society and recreate an entirely new one on new/modern/progressive principles. In each case, the children and the youth were seen as the hope for the future; those growing up were least tainted by the evils of the previous society. The Sabra, children brought up on the Kibbutz, were the personification of cherished ideals of many, not just in Israel. The revolutionaries in Russia established their Young Pioneers and gave priority to youth. The Hitler Youth were to underpin the Reich which would last a thousand years. The idealization of youth is common in times that identify themselves as progressive, but such worship of youth is not necessarily associated with lack of discipline and authority.

Riley (1988) also draws attention to the failure of modern Western societies to provide suitable roles appropriate for the growing numbers of elderly people. William Ogburn's (1964) concept of "cultural lag" seeks to explain the phenomenon of changes in social institutions and popular philosophy falling behind technology and economic advance. Riley suggests this has a recent counterpart in the concept of "structural age" (Riley et al. 1988a), as outmoded social institutions fail to provide opportunities for the growing aspirations and increased numbers of older people. This idea, while superficially having merit, is open to the standard critique of all similar modernization theories, because it views social change as taking a particular inevitable course. Such views tend to lead towards complacency; they assume there is an automatic process which corrects these social inadequacies, as ideas and social institutions "catch up". In contrast, the political economy view is that rather than "outmoded institutions" being the problem, it is the construction of new structures of oppression that needs to be examined. It is not that old people experience inequality because they cannot overthrow the expectations of the past, it is that their current lives are being positively and continually structured by current institutions.

Peter Laslett (1989) in his writing on the Third Age has formulated this problem more coherently. He sees cultural change lagging behind demographic change. The ageing of populations, which has gone on for some time (in Britain at least since 1911), has expanded the older age groups in society, but no new roles have developed to give meaning to these expanded demographic groups. He sees the problem of the Third Age as a cultural one; the need to develop and give meaning to the last third of life. This formulation of the problem is more historically accurate, but the excellent historical demography must not lull us into the view that cultures are either inherently inflexible or not closely tied into the social and demographic fabric of society. Any failure on the part of society to change its cultural evaluation of old age requires explanation just as much as any continuity in values.

Simone de Beauvoir's (1972) classic exposition of the double jeopardy of being old and female also serves to illustrate how interconnected cultural constructions of undervalued social groups are. The twin cultural processes, first of individualism, and secondly of appearances, spectacle and display, connect in the fetishism of body image. The growth of individualism has been linked to growth in rationality and systematization of social life, to the experience of urban life, to the requirements of modern labour processes, to secularization, and to the development of modern welfare systems. Its development is a core subject for sociology. The extent to which people encounter each other through transient social relationships, and experience each other, not through interaction and dialogue, but as receivers and transmitters of mass images, appearance and display, becomes crucial. Social knowledge of other people becomes limited to their appearance. Reflexively, we come to regard who we are to be more closely tied to what we look like. The great spread of such depressive illnesses as bulimia and anorexia has been associated with adolescent girls in particular because it occurs at a time crucial to the establishment of an independent adult personality, which in our society has become tightly linked to body image (Turner 1984, Featherstone 1982, Giddens 1991). At the other end of the age span, loss of adult status and body image are also closely linked. Failure to maintain an acceptable body image, a desirable appearance, is a problem for both men and women in old age. Men in later life, however, tend to have access to other desirable images through displays of wealth and power, which women do not. This last point should alert us to the need, not only to note how important body image is to status, but also to consider the relationship between culture and ideology, and ask *how* and *why* particular images come to be valued.

It is possible to mount a critique of the approach to the inequality in old age as the loss of cultural value, old age as a roleless role, the fag end of life lacking the charisma of youth, from a straightforward materialist perspective drawn from the kind of data presented in the comparative analysis of old age across different societies presented in Chapter 3. Positive images of old age derive from elderly people with access to power; the patriarchs and matriarchs of extended families, where kinship and family labour give power, are seen as self-confident, handsome and respected. Where spiritual authority confirms power on older people, the body form of those possessing power does not diminish it. Such power may well be seen to shine through their eyes, or be self-evident in their serene demeanour. In order to understand what is happening in our society, we need to look at how the changing material basis of the life course interacts with the cultural construction of the meaning of life-course transitions. We need to examine at least the possibility that old people are stereotyped as unattractive because they lack property and power, rather than the converse.

The despiritualized striving for personal perfection, particularly of body image, is typical of social values in late twentieth-century Western society. This despiritualized striving is related to the Protestant Ethic argument, whereby the individual striving to represent the ideal of God's chosen elect is transformed into a secularized version of the value of striving to achieve work and entrepreneurial ideals for their own sake, independently of the material satisfactions or consumer pleasures success might bring. In the contemporary West, the despiritualized striving shifts from a work career to personal self-fulfilment. At the extreme this can manifest itself as a dedicated hedonism, the relentless pursuit of extremes of sensation, perhaps through drugs or the adrenaline flush of soccer aggro, perhaps justified as the systematic widening of personal experience and thus moving further down the road to self-knowledge and self-fulfilment. This is reflected in the deification of a particular notion of love in contemporary Western culture. Love is defined as a sensation felt between two people, and its supreme sacrament is the sexual act – preferably a mutual orgasm. In practice, personal fulfilment becomes a series of highly fragmented obsessions; from assembling the finest stamp collection, to achieving perfect breast size, from achieving the outstanding educational success of one's children to acquiring the most stunning hairstyle, from perfectly manicured nails to writing the definitive book on old age. Personal self-fulfilment defined in this way becomes problematic for people near the end of their life course. This is because of a paradox that is based around the fact that the ideal of self-fulfilment is never achievable, it is the striving itself that gives the value to life within this set of cultural values, and hence those nearest the end of that striving are confronted with the impossibility and futility of further striving.

Thus, although Laslett and Greer are right to point to the cultural problem of constructing a meaningful old age in our society, they are both wrong as to the origins of the problem. Greer is wrong to make inappropriate generalizations from the specific experience of a particular cohort – particularly the one of which she is a member. Laslett is wrong in that he underestimates the rapidity of cultural change and does not explore in sufficient depth how such cultural adaptation takes place. It is not that old age roles are an unchanging social residual, and that the numbers of these residual people have got larger, rather the residuality of old people is actively and continually re-created in our society.

The call for increased respect for parents and the reassertion of parental authority will make no difference to the social role of elderly people. Such a change in values and behaviour is unachievable without change in the social causes of the perceived lack of power and authority for parents. To lament the rise of individualism is not to change it. It is important to distinguish power and authority from love and respect. Social surveys continue to show love, respect, loyalty and the strength of family affection between generations (Finch 1989, Wenger 1984, Minkler 1991). This is not the same as accepting the authority of senior generations to direct behaviour and the power to enforce their will on the younger generation. The rapidity of social and economic change, and of social and geographical mobility, has among many other factors rendered such power ineffective.

What might be required is a positive re-evaluation of some aspects of history and tradition that strengthen the sources of value and status of elderly people. One way in which elderly people have become undervalued is that their economic skill and knowledge have been rendered obsolete by technical and organizational change. However, as environmental limits are drawn tighter and tighter around the expansion of material consumption and the methods of mass production, old knowledge and skills might well need to be revalued. There has been such a revitalization of some traditional and folk medical knowledge; alternative or complementary medicine has an increasing popularity. Independent of the efficacy or the reasons for its popularity, those who remember the traditional practices and recipes and how to prepare them can gain respect and status. This is also true of craft and domestic skills. However, it has to be recognized that two centuries of rationalization, and secularization, accompanied by the bureaucratization, and professionalization of knowledge, make such reversal highly problematic. Doctors are not readily going to relinquish their power to define and control death (Turner 1987); and if they did, this role would most likely fall into the even more dubious hands of the lawyers.

A further problem with the argument that identifies the problem of old age roles as their residual or left-over quality is an insufficient attention to the issues of globalization. Societal ageing has been going on in Europe for a considerable time and is still largely identified as a European issue (Czechoslovak Demographic Society 1989). Although, in fact, other world populations are also ageing, and indeed ageing faster than Europe, they have not yet reached the proportion of the population currently experienced in the West. Thus because of both the predominance of West European cultures in the world through the global history of colonialism and the fact that it is Europeans who have identified the ageing of populations as a problem, analyses of the issue tend to be highly Euro-centric. This

Euro-centrism gives cause for both hope and concern: hope, because other cultures might, translated to the West, create valued and respected roles relevant for elderly people; concern, because continued Westernization may undermine the position of elderly people across the world. Indeed, the association of the demographically ageing populations with the ex-colonial and imperial powers, and the new developing economies with large expanding young populations, may create an, as yet, unexplored source of concern and tension.

One response to ageism has been systematic attempts to produce positive images of elderly people. There have been numbers of books that have given pictorial or autobiographical images of outstanding and successful elderly people (Comfort 1977). A new talent for writing or painting discovered when over eighty; marathon runners of similar age; television programmes showing us exciting, stimulating, quick-witted, interesting 90-year-olds, these image-building attempts are to be applauded and do have positive effects, particularly in those aspects of ageism that become internalized and self-limiting. However, such attempts contain a problem. They most frequently present people as successfully retaining "youthful" attributes. In other words, such image-building does not revalue the category "old" in itself, rather it encourages the possibility of extending youth (Friedan 1993). This is revealed in the necessity of, after having invented the Third Age, having to invent the Fourth Age. The Third Age can be a time of growth, new horizons and new possibilities or self-fulfilment. However, at some point in their lives individuals experience a physical decline prior to death; for some it may last a long time, for many others it will be mercifully short. Hence, having conceptualized the Third Age as a life stage defined by the possibilities of growth, and as death and physical decline are inevitable, a further stage – a Fourth Age of growing dependency – is required to retain the integrity of the idea. The Third Age movement has had a tremendously positive effect on the lifestyles of retired people. However, although it has revised images of retirement, it has not been able to challenge the cultural meaning of old age *per se*.

There are two possibilities that lead to crucially different attitudes and policies when addressing this issue of the cultural evaluation of old age. Either, what is required is a reduction in the salience of age-based roles and images (for example, the use of a walking stick or the latest "street cred" fashions being in no sense incongruous on a person of the "wrong" age). Bytheway (1995) makes a strong argument that overcoming ageism requires that age becomes socially irrelevant. Or, what is needed is a positive image of old age (for example, a cultural equation of age with wisdom; nobody under 70 years of age has seen enough of life to make sound judgements). Those who identify postmodern trends in contemporary society would anticipate that the first scenario is more probable than the second.

CHAPTER FIVE

Social theories of inequality: gender, race, class and age

How have social scientists sought to understand social differentiation and social inequality and to what extent do these theories make sense when applied to the condition of elderly people? This chapter seeks to provide a major critique of existing theories of inequality as partial and limited. By examining the theories that have sought to explain the inequalities associated with class, gender and ethnicity, the need for a general theory that will encompass all inequalities, including that of age, is revealed (Brodkin 1989). It is necessary to emphasize the *processes* of inequality and not merely to multiply the categories of disadvantage. Insufficient work has been done in theorizing the relationship of age to society (Johnson 1978). Significantly, two recent major undergraduate textbooks that seek to make comprehensive analyses of British society in the 1980s simply fail to discuss old age and elderly people (Abercrombie & Ward 1988, McDowell et al. 1989). The discussion of these issues is much further advanced in the United States where sociologists, anthropologists and historians have made significant contributions about the ways in which we might think about these issues. Nancy Foner has attempted an anthropological study of old age and inequality, which brings together some excellent and interesting material particularly on the position of older women across a range of societies and in the role of the supernatural in the power and control elderly people can exert (Foner 1984). Foner deals with the issues within the traditional boundaries of anthropological subject matter, while my project is rather larger and rather more risky. My argument is that, in order to understand adequately the issue of inequality and old age, our theoretical under-standing of inequality itself needs to be revised and systematized, and it needs to incorporate a broader humanistic conception of human beings. We need to avoid compartmentalizing people's experience of inequality and think in terms of a historical changing society made up of a variety of interconnected life-long human experiences.

There is, of course, no ready agreement as to the nature of inequal-ity. Some see inequality primarily as a function of power and wealth. Thus inequality is looked at as a product of social and economic insti-tutions. To change towards a society that is more equal between men and women, between ethnic groups and between classes requires a change in the political and economic structure of society. For others inequality is at root a feature of culture, and manifest in the values systems and symbols of sexism, racism and ageism, and such that some sections of society are subject to invidious evaluation and nega-tive stereotyping. What is required for a more equal society is seen from this point of view as the re-education of dominant groups, a re-evaluation of disadvantaged groups and a cultural reassertion by those who have been labelled as unequal. Naturally writers have tried to understand inequality within a framework that can contain both social-structural and cultural perspectives but, in practice, most have given one priority over the other. Weber's distinction between class and status reflects the cultural/structural opposition: social status derives from social honour – the esteem and evaluation society places on a social position; whereas class is the product of the market position which sets of actors occupy. The decline in the critical impact of Marxism has much to do with its relegation of issues of race and gender to the lesser category of status distinctions while class issues are given analytical priority. Some argue that power structures are so strong and/or cultural images so dominant that only radical separation can provide a route to greater equality. Ethnic or racial groups must break away and form their own nations and have their own territory; women must distance themselves from men and create their own institutions and culture; class can only be overcome in new separate communitarian societies, as in the Kibbutz, New Lanarkshire or Walden. I make this point to emphasize that theory is not a purely abstract activity; it is a guide to action. Without a theory of inequality it is not possible to think what, if any-thing, to do about it. The most helpful approach to these issues is to stick closely to the specifics of people's experience and not over-reify abstract dichotomies such as culture/social structure or cling on to them too tenaciously when their analytical usefulness is past. "We might also take seriously Dewey's suggestion that the way to re-enchant the world, to bring back what religion gave our forefathers, is to stick to the concrete." (Rorty 1994: 170) It is not in the abstract that inequality and old age need to be re-evaluated, we are most likely to learn most from the practical reasoning of those struggling directly with these problems. I will deal with the issues of gender, race and class (in that order), not with a comprehensive survey but selecting those ideas most pertinent to inequality and old age.

Natural categories

Old age seems "natural" but it is nevertheless a social construction (Hazan 1994). Ageing is a biological process that happens to all of us from the moment we are born. It is a continuous process. It has features in common with, and differences from, both sex-based categories and those differences in appearance that become labelled as "race". Some societies attach social significance to particular phenotypical variations and these are sometimes labelled as racial differences; for example, the meaning attached to skin colour varies across the world (Banton 1983). All societies have some form of gender role differentiation based conceptually on sexual difference. Some societies assign social significance to aspects of appearance and behaviour that are thought of as biologically determined indicators of age. The three categories, "age", "gender" and "race", are sometimes called "natural categories". This is said to be because they indicate social roles on the basis of natural or biologically determined differences between human beings. However, it is crucial to keep in mind the difference between the sign and what is being signified by the sign. The profile of the figure on the toilet door is no guarantee of the shape of the ceramic ware behind it. Apparently biological cues do not tell us anything socially significant about people without a cultural framework of interpretation.

Because they appear to be "natural", these signs are sometimes seen as universal. The imputed universality of such roles, however, lies in the assumed biologically universal occurrence of such phenomena not in their meaning or significance. It is a social process that establishes whether skin pigmentation, wrinkles or hair have any meaning in a particular social situation, and what that meaning might be. Just as studies of racial ideologies and typifications have shown that ethnic symbols are not fixed in biology, so has the feminist contribution to sociology shown how gender is socially constructed. Thus in some societies women are seen as emotional intuitive types of people, in others they are hard-headed or practical. The reverse pattern is also true, in some societies it is men who are labelled emotional – easily moved to tears; on the other hand they may be seen as hard-headed, practical creatures. "Natural" has connotations other than the biological, that of being obvious – without question. It also frequently stands for "normal" in a moral sense as for example when used in terms of sexuality.

Many of the cues that are used to allocate people into the categories men or women, old or young, black or white, although biological in origin, only have significance because they are selected by a social process which attributes meaning to them. Those cues which become selected and socially recognized come to have conventional meanings to a set of people. The potential number of such cues is very large indeed and only a very limited number emerge from the historical social process and become meaningful. The culturally defined content of age-based statuses also varies from culture to culture and over history. These age categories are like the other "natural" categories in the sociological literature and also seen as "natural" in both the sense of given in nature (i.e. determined by biology) and being obvious (i.e. taken for granted or common sense). In each society there is some degree of phasing of life course and some ways of behaving are more or less appropriate depending on how old you are; it is a taken-for-granted part of social life that you have to "act your age".

Evolutionary arguments, used by those who attempt socio-biological accounts of "natural" inequality, tend to have the characteristics of *post hoc* reconstructions, explaining how things have to be like they are because they are like they are (Sanderson 1990). Such quasi evolutionary explanations are not explanations of particular patterns of variation in human social behaviour, they give rationalizations of generalized universal patterns. The logical problem with this approach is that they are teleological explanations based on the consequences not the origins of a phenomenon. These social biology theories also have an empirical problem of moving from evolution in pre-history to particular modern societies. Suggesting that grand-mother nurturing has survival value for an altruistic gene in the late Pleistocene era, scarcely goes a long way to explaining why histori-cally women retire at 60 in Britain rather than 65 (as do men), and why this was changed in 1994. To many it is comforting to know that older women rather than the male killer apes have been the driv-ing force in human evolution (Dahlberg 1981, Lee & DeVore 1968). But why then are elderly women held in such low esteem in so many contemporary societies? It is not possible to progress from these evolutionary and socio-biological theories to developing explanations of the changing role of grandparents, or other features of old age, in contemporary society. Such evolutionary arguments tell us very little about current gender relationships, and can equally tell us little about age-based relationships. However, the problems of explaining female post-fertile longevity is a cautionary tale about paying atten-tion to the whole life course and the interplay between generations when understanding social behaviour even within the social biology paradigm.

Gender as a model for age inequality

How are the inequalities associated with gender both similar and dif-ferent from those experienced by people on the basis of age? There has been a great deal written over the last twenty years, and some significant progress made, on understanding women's role in society and on analysing the oppression of women. It will be impossible within the confines of this book to review all the existing ideas in gender studies applicable to the theme of age-based inequality. How-ever, some theories are extremely suggestive of how the social pro-cess of ageism operates very much like that of sexism. In a similar vein there is a considerable literature that has looked at issues of rac-ism and ethnicity, which may also provide insights into ageism. The parallels and contrasts between ageism and sexism and racism are discussed in a growing literature (Bytheway 1995, McEwen 1990). There have been studies that have looked at the gender divisions within the older community, and others that have looked at the position of ethnic minority elders (Arber & Ginn 1991, Askham et al. 1993). My purpose is to look the other way around and see if explanations of inequality derived from race and from gender can illuminate the inequality experienced by older people in general.

Some anthropologists have sought to give cultural accounts of gender inequality. Cultural analyses attempt to identify processes in thought or in communication which influence the use of symbols and the performance of culture. Sherry Ortner's (1974) view of the cultural origin of the devaluation of the female gender starts from the dichotomy between nature and culture. Structuralists from Lévi-Strauss onwards have discussed the importance of this opposition and its transformations because it lies at the root of how social life explains itself and establishes what is social and what is not. Thus culture is the positive category and nature, as the unsocial opposite, has negative connotations. If society is not to be overwhelmed by the wild, powerful, untamed forces of nature, then culture must be able to impose a significant meaningful order on it. Ortner suggests that women are seen as more "natural" than men. The "earth mother" gives birth, has extended reproductive functions and breasts that produce milk, menstruates and thus can be thought of as less amenable to cultural rules than male bodies with their limited role in reproduction. From this stems the structural logic of the constructs –

female:nature::male:culture.

Ortner's position suggests the devaluation of the female gender is a product of the structure of culture itself; its universality comes from the imperatives of the construction of cultural life.

Is it possible to apply a similar logic to that of Ortner's gender argument to the position of elderly people and the use of age criteria in society? Is there a parallel cultural structure in the social categorization of age and the culture:nature opposition? Children, especially small children, are seen as natural and not fully social, so do not have the same rights and statuses as fully acculturated adults. In so far as elderly people are sometimes treated as infants, in particular when they show signs of infirmity and cannot impose the necessary social restraints on their bodily functions, then they may also be thought of as closer to nature (Hockey & James 1993). Hence the structure Ortner identifies also locates the old and the young in the natural realm as opposed to the cultural status of the adult. The logic of the cultural devaluation argument for gender is also applicable to the case of age.

However, the distinction between nature and culture is itself a cultural construct (Strathern 1980). What is considered to be "natural" in one context can be considered "cultural" in another. Both with age and gender, the universal pattern is more apparent than real. Peggy Reeves Sanday (1981) argues that there is a variety of mythical scripts for explaining the relative social patterns of power and dominance between genders. These myths can be understood as stories implying statements about moral order and thus depending on the distinguishing of cultural rule from natural disorder. However, Sanday explains the variety of myth and the changing patterns of dominance through material relations and environmental crises. Male violence is sometimes one "solution" adopted when societies are confronted with stressful conditions. Similarly it is possible to argue that, as with gender, the changing evaluation of age also needs to be seen in the context of changing material crises and stresses in society. There are cultural processes by which people come to understand and express these changes, myths and categories are retold and redrawn to make sense of the changing circumstances.

Negative body images

The social reproduction of gender images has been a concern of feminist literature. The examination and analysis of the way women have been portrayed in the media, magazines, television, literature and other cultural forms has been a central part of women's studies. The manipulation of these images is seen as a major way in which women are oppressed and conditioned into particular views of themselves and their bodies. Parallel arguments can be advanced for the experience of elderly people. The often repeated experience of older people of belated shocked recognition of themselves as the elderly image they glimpse in the shop window illustrates the distance between the internalized body image and the exterior reality. Many stigmatized groups come to think of their physical characteristics as different from those which others see as theirs. The social pressures to conform to appropriate styles, behaviour and body image that have affected women also affect the elderly. Indeed elderly women are in a particularly oppressed position (Sontag 1978). Similarities exist between sexist language and images and ageist language and images:

for example, the picture postcard humour stereotypes the buxom blonde, the fat wife and the toothless lecher. Simone de Beauvoir (1972) was characteristically sharp in exposing the double jeopardy experienced by older women.

External images have become more valued than internal images of beauty or virtue. Those whose exteriors do not conform to aesthetic standards as body objects are valued less, and come to value themselves less. Internal characteristics of virtue, wisdom or spirituality have become less respected. The translation of "grace" from a spiritual characteristic to a method of comportment is an indicative example. In recent years, in the West, the aesthetic standards of body image have become thinner and more muscular and more concentrated on bodies rather than faces. The development of these aesthetic judgements both as to body shape and exteriority have documented histories, they develop out of pre-existing values and judgements (Giddens 1991).

Ageism, like sexism and racism, is embedded in the rules and structures of society. However, all these are based not only in institutions but also in cultural stereotypes. These stereotypes, just like the institutions, are rooted in history. An understanding of both the social structural processes and the cultural processes underpinning the development of negative stereotypes is required. Thus the decline in status of the elderly in the West is associated with secularization and medicalization of old age (Kirk 1992), and can be seen as devaluing death and old age as mundane and potentially controllable natural processes, i.e. recategorized from high status culture to low status nature. However, this analysis of how the devaluation was achieved needs to be interrelated with the processes of industrialization, urbanization and the development of capitalism which produced powerful secular and professional institutions.

While these discussions on the reproduction of the sexist or ageist images are an interesting and necessary part of the debate, as is the examination of their internal symbolic structures, the essential theoretical task of explaining origins and variation is not encompassed by studies that count nipples and wrinkles in a given text and seek merely to document the extent of sexism or ageism. It seems to me a more important task to discover *why* negative body images of elderly people prevail as opposed to discovering *how* the negative evaluation is achieved (McNay 1992).

Age and female roles in the division of labour

Patriarchy is one of the most common concepts used to attempt to explain female subordination. The idea is frequently seen as a universal condition of male power over women and is variously associated with violence, sex, marriage and the family (Walby 1990). The essential feature of patriarchy is to locate women's oppression within the institution of the family. Originally the concept of patriarchy referred to rule not by men but by fathers (Turner 1984: 155). The patriarchal extended family classically consists of: father (as head of the household), wife, sons, their wives, their children and any unmarried daughters. Thus patriarchy includes not only domination on the basis of gender but domination on the basis of age. The patriarch is in authority over not only his wife but his children even when they are adult and irrespective of their sex. Further, in some patriarchal extended families it is the elder brother, in the absence of the father, who dominates the household including his younger brothers. Age is significant in ordering social relationships within a patriarchal household, not only between the patriarch and others but for example between the inmarrying women; the most immediate oppression felt by junior wives is most frequently that of their mother-in-law. This is because she is likely to be in charge of the new wife in the day-to-day work and ensures the newcomer fulfils her responsibilities to the new household she has joined. Thus the patriarchal extended family is structured by both age and gender (Goody 1990). How much of the discussion of patriarchy in the context of gender subordination can be transferred directly to the discussion of age-based inequality?

The major problem with many discussions of patriarchy, illuminating as they are about conditions of inequality, is that they posit universal social characteristics. Theories of the devaluation of the female gender by men, in which patriarchy is seen as a universal social condition, are, as a result, ineffective in explaining the variation in gender relations and thus in suggesting ways of changing them. If we want to understand how gender relations in the modern world are changing, and how they differ from other societies and previous times, we need theories that account for the range of inequalities and relationships. The really interesting ideas are those that explain why inequality varies, for example theories that attempt to explain why women's domestic labour is rigorously exploited in some societies but remains relatively untrammelled by men in others (Boserup 1970). Similarly, it is the range of age-based inequalities that we wish to understand and not simply to assert (incorrectly) that all elderly people are devalued. The enormous variety of gender relations found across the range of human societies suggests that cultural explanations that describe social processes of the construction of inequality are required. The same logic must also apply to the variety of age-based relationships.

A further key idea is that of "domestication" of women: the restriction of female roles to private family and household worlds. The economic subordination of women can reflect both the aspects of gender relations; the exploitation of female labour can be seen as part of the patriarchal relationship including the "unproductive" (unpaid) home servicing that directly supports male "productive"(paid) work. One set of arguments that seeks to explain the historical development of patriarchy locates the origins and nature of women's subordination in the development of sexual divisions of labour and private property.

> The sexual division of labour emerges as an expression of women's roles in both production and reproduction; these roles in turn derive from those social relations that regulate the formation of families and the bearing and rearing of children, and those social relations that govern the production of goods and services. (Deere et al. 1982, quoted in Momson & Townsend 1987: 66)

Engels' (1884) *The origins of the family, private property and the state* is the starting point of many of these discussions. The gender division of labour was the first division of labour (although age-based divisions must be close behind). Explaining the origin of the division of labour is crucial to understanding not only gender inequalities but the development of human society with all its inequalities. Many see the dominance of modern capitalism as the result of the most successful method of organizing a highly complex division of labour yet seen. Engels' essential point is that there was a historical development from communal egalitarian societies through the rise of private property and the family to exploitive class societies. He held the erroneous Victorian evolutionary sequence of initial human promiscuity, followed by matriarchy and then patriarchy. What is useful, however, is the theory of the mechanism of change. In his view, women became subordinate with the appearance of means of production that could be privately owned. The domestication of plants and animals enabled land and stock to, potentially, become private property. When men held private property rights in productive assets that produced an exchangeable surplus, women's labour could be exploited. Thus women came to work for their husbands and families instead of for society. Other exploitive relationships could develop from this start, which included: slave and master, lord and serf, capitalist and worker. With the rise of capitalism, production and reproduction became separated, the home was no longer also the workplace.

One key exploitive mechanism is the process by which women's unpaid domestic labour becomes the social effort which the owners of capital need to create the next generation of the workforce. By not paying for that reproduction of the workforce, and because wages are set by supply and demand not the costs in effort of reproducing labour, then employers are able to command a larger share of the social product at the expense of women. Women's unpaid domestic work is used to cheapen the value of labour as a commodity. What needs to be added to this analysis is that elders are part of the domestic sphere of production and reproduction. They, like women, were separated from productive roles by the industrial division of labour and they too play a role in reproductive activity in the broad sense of creating the next generations for society. This observation will become important again when discussing the issue of generation equity which is discussed later in connection with the redistributive role of pension schemes. The key point is that the productive capacity of the younger generation depends on the work, activity and investment of the senior generation.

Wright (1985) identifies a number of mechanisms by which resources in contemporary society come to be differentially allocated between men and women. Some or all of the wage differentials between men and women, he suggests, can be attributed directly to the distribution of skill and organizational assets between men and women. Gender relations constitute one mechanism that helps to explain the distribution of resources, such as valued skills and strategic social positions, which enable some people to obtain greater rewards for their work than others. Gender itself could, Wright argues, be conceived of as a special kind of credential that works in the same way as other monopolization of skills and position through credentially regulated barriers. These barriers structure market and labour relationships and so create exploitation. Sex segregation of occupations may function in a parallel way by confining women to certain categories of jobs thus reducing the competition in other jobs held by men (Crompton & Sanderson 1990).

The same argument, which identifies a natural category as a job credential and therefore something that structures access to labour markets, can also be applied to age and elderly people. These arguments extended to the condition of old age would suggest that we should look for processes by which elders, and indeed young people, are excluded from skill acquisition and power positions by use of age-based credentials. "Buggins turn" promotions or compulsory retirement ages would be examples of such exclusionary processes. Not only are there formal age requirements for acquisition of many jobs, there are also compulsory retirement ages and age-based exclusionary processes even for those in employment. This is reflected in the increasing difficulty that those made unemployed later in life have in finding work.

Wright's second analytical thrust comes from debating how housewives relate to the class structure. Wives of male workers providing their husbands with domestic services may be seen as working class because they are indirectly exploited by capital through their contribution to the subsistence of their husbands. Alternatively housewives may be seen to occupy a position in the subsistence or domestic mode of production and can thus be seen as exploited by their husbands within that subsidiary class relation. Some writers have argued that the concept of class simply does not pertain to those outside the labour force and thus housewives are not in any class at all. Where women are chattels of their husband or father and simply by virtue of their gender have a specific place within the social relations of production then they constitute a class. Certain radical feminists maintain that women are a class but they claim that this is the universal condition of women and are not simply claiming that under a special historical condition this may happen. Class is not equivalent to oppression. Such a wide use of the term "class" is not very helpful because it abandons a key analytical tool for identifying a precise form of inequality produced by the relationship of exploitation found in a historically specific form of society.

Clearly there are parallels in the position of elderly people who are co-residents with others and make the kinds of contribution to a domestic economy as are made by a housewife. Indeed studies show that close proximate residence often has the effect of increased grandparental support for child care, domestic duties and financial aid; a common household is not necessary for a flow of labour and resources down the generations. The complex flow of resources between members of households, kin, neighbours and friends, has been examined empirically but such exchanges have seldom been placed comprehensively within the broader political economy (Qureshi & Walker 1989). We can take forward to our discussion of age-based inequality the question as to whether elderly people who are outside of the workforce, and outside of familial and domestic arrangements, have any class position. Given that some of the poorest people in our society are elderly women living on their own, they should be central to an analysis of inequality. I do not think that social theories that exclude such people's contribution to society as unproductive and fail to recognize the exploitation they experience through their life course are a helpful way forward. It is precisely in understanding the interplay between such conditions as class and gender that the concept of life course can start to come into its own. Class and gender have been key forces shaping the life courses of elder women and thus the position of social inequality they currently occupy.

Age, ethnicity and nationalism

Because sociology is essentially about group formation, the issue of ethnicity and identity is at the heart of the subject. How do groups of people identify themselves as "us" – a sense of being one and the same; as opposed to "them" – those different others. A full understanding of ethnicity thus requires a skill that sociologists have not yet reliably achieved, which is the successful combination of structural type arguments and phenomenological type arguments. That is to say, we need to bring together how people see and think about their own and other groups with how those groups fit together as part of some social order. There are at least three major strands in the intellectual endeavour which has sought to understand the issue of ethnicity. The differences between these strands reflect not only historical traditions within academic life but also different theoretical starting points. First there is the view that ethnic groups are historically continuous specific social groups. In this view, to be a proper ethnic group the claims in the group's myth of origin must have an authentic historical reality that is rooted in a long past and is thus linked with biological reproduction and continuity. In this view, the biological group is real and the symbols of ethnicity merely express that pre-existing difference. The second and contrary view sees ethnicity as highly malleable, having different meanings at different times and places. That which creates ethnicity is the socially defined boundary that identifies the difference between "them" and "us". From this point of view the reality of the boundary in the sense of historical or biological continuity is irrelevant. It is the use to which the social construction of difference is put that matters. Hence ethnicities can be born and disappear, and can also be situationally contingent, i.e. some markers of difference only appear in certain kinds of social situation and are not relevant to others. The difference in names between Serbs and Croats, so important in the Balkans, is both invisible and irrelevant in Britain. A third view of ethnicity is that it is born out of conflict. The structure of society and economy created differing interests and people come to express and articulate these conflicts in a variety of ways including racialism and ethnic rivalry. From this view the conflicts of interest are real but the cultural and symbolic formulation of those conflicts might not accurately reflect them (Rex & Mason 1986, Miles 1982).

There is a debate in the literature on race relations that has not always been very productive that attempts to distinguish between race and ethnicity. I tend to agree with Wallman (1978) that race must be regarded as one among many forms of ethnicity because it is not the phenotypical marker itself, i.e. skin colour, nose shape, height or whatever, which matters but the social significance of such markers. Further social cues such as language, dress and religion can also play a role in creating differences that are colloquially labelled "racial", even though they are learnt not inherited behaviour. To differentiate one kind of social marker from another is to concretize and over-rigidify social boundaries. However, race/ethnicity is more than simply boundary marking, it is a process of group formation (and dissolution) and these groups can have long and powerful historical traditions. Or perhaps more accurately, large and powerful ethnic groups can claim long historical traditions. Anthony D. Smith (1981) tends to over-concretize ethnic categories but does point out their historical evolution. His main contribution is to point out the association between modernization and the search for community that creates the cyclical dynamic of ethnic revival. We can take from this discussion the idea of age, like ethnicity, as a historically developing (but socially derived and thus plastic) social category that is variable both in content and in coverage.

In what kinds of circumstance are the "them" and "us" likely to refer to age-based categories? Clearly they cannot refer to "ethne" in Smith's (1981) strong sense of ethnic group, as they can never be historically continuous, biological, reproducing groups. However, certain distinctions based on age can be made to seem more fundamental, important and inviolable by acquiring ancient provenance and long pedigree and thus become sanctified by tradition. The social constructionist perspective appears to have considerable relevance to understanding the changing salience of age-based roles. Those societies that seek to institutionalize ethnic distinction must socially, usually bureaucratically, organize the boundary; for example, require religion to be visible (e.g. to display the Star of David) or to enact legislation that defines what degree of descent taints the blood for enslavement, or operate pass laws that register those allowed access to public facilities. So, by a similar social logic, societies that institutionalize age distinction also require the birth certificate, the student card or the bus pass. Further, in modern impersonal urban settings, where interaction takes place in the absence of the mutual knowledge that is characteristic of small communities, social badges and markers take on added significance; in the absence of other knowledge, stereotypes based on ethnicity, or for that matter age, have to substitute for personal familiarity.

Ethnic conspiracy theories and the language of conflict

The language of ethnicity or nationalism is part of a system of thought that is closed, circular and rigid. The ethnic conspiracy explanation for personal troubles always works and can seldom be discredited. In situations of conflict it provides a ready-made language of abuse to relieve guilt and tension and blame the other party. In a traffic accident the other driver is not berated as "you stupid Skoda driver" or "you tall thin idiot", it is as "you black bastard", or "bog paddy" or "Serbian peasant/fascist Croat". In parallel, the more aggressive ageist stereotypes can be brought up in situations of conflict.

Faced with one of the many bureaucratic organization problems that beset life in modern state societies, finding a job, getting a pension, obtaining permission to build a house, etc. are examples of where racism/ethnic nationalism comes to be expressed. The belief in the ethnic conspiracy – they help their own, the only way to get things done is personal contact – becomes in practice ethnic favouritism. People naturally maximize their opportunities when they negotiate with such bureaucracies. They do it the official way – fill in forms, make applications, but they also do it the unofficial way – ring up who they know, use personal networks to offer inducements and ask favours. If the application works, even if it was legitimate and would have worked anyway, the ethnic conspiracy is confirmed. If the application fails, the ethnic conspiracy also explains the situation. The applicants may rationalize to themselves that the contacts were not powerful enough, the "others" got in the way and did "us" down. Again looked at from the alternative ethnicity, this application and its outcome are also explicable in terms of ethnic conspiracy. The success of the application was ethnic favouritism. Its failure was because the application was not valid anyway and thus it is only right that the applicants were refused and they are only aggrieved because they have an ethnic chip on their shoulder. In other words, whatever happens – to the general public, applicants, potential applicants and other observers – the most consistent explanation is ethnic favouritism. The bureaucrats and officials doing the administration, because however objectively they do their job people still think ethnic advantage is being given, will find it very difficult not to confirm to this expectation. If age-based conflict ever did come about I am confident that a similar conspiracy for and against the age groups would also arise. It is the absence of such language and conspiratorial explanations that suggests such conflict does not currently exist.

What is the relationship between gender, ethnicity and age as a method of generating social inequality? We need to understand how these inequalities intersect to create the distinctive life-course opportunities that for example mean that older black women get a rough deal when society's wealth is shared out. Some writers have argued that some of these forms of inequality are more significant than others. The view that all oppression is ultimately class based is one such point of view. However, others have sought to try and understand the interrelationships between the various forms of inequality (Dressel 1991). As we shall see later in this book, some writers have argued that there are real conflicts of interests between different age groups in contemporary society. However, they see these conflicts as being hidden and not fully expressed in the political, legal or other conflict arenas. This is the reverse of the argument made by those who see ethnic conflicts as displaced economic interests. Ethnic groups, as with gender and age groups, may have common interests, but these are specific and contingent on particular historical developments in specific times and places. They do not have a more general significance; it is not possible to tell *a priori* if such conflicts are likely or inevitable. What such theories do suggest is that when looking at new constructions of social identity, including those based on age, it is sensible to look at the variety of new interests being expressed (and indeed at groups who are not overt players in the action but whose interests might nevertheless be involved).

Age, exploitation and complex class relationships

If class is defined in terms of employment, work or the division of labour, what does class mean, if anything, post-retirement? The position of elderly people in the social division of labour needs to be adequately understood and key concepts like exploitation, life-chances and interests need to be reassessed from the "life-course" perspective. In the early 1970s Harris put forward a thesis that ageing is a process of deprivation: "In terms of both income and employment, the old are deprived relative both to the rest of society and relative to their previous life experiences, but that this deprivation is mediated by the class structure, magnifying it at the bottom and minimising it at the top." (Harris 1975, quoted in Phillipson & Walker 1986: 21)

Class is clearly crucial to understanding inequality in modern society. If we ask the question "Is disadvantage in old age a feature of class?" then we must not answer this question as if the disadvantaged class are those who are exploited through wage labour. Classes are usually thought of as social groups with common interests, they are the result of the way in which the modern productive system known as capitalism organizes the division of labour and regulates access to what is produced. Therefore if we limit the idea of classes strictly to those who have common interests in the labour market, this deprives retired people of a class. From a particular, limited, economistic perspective, retired people have differing interests from those in wage employment, retired people as consumers have interests in low prices and thus low labour costs. In what sense might elderly people be thought of as exploited? An unreconstructed Marxist approach might see them as living off the production/surplus value generated by workers. To obtain a full understanding it is necessary to view class within a life-course perspective. Such a long-term view might, for example, see workers bargaining with employers for current wages but also for pensions as deferred wages (Achenbaum 1983), and thus also identify, for example, differing preferences within organized labour between older and younger workers in the balance between current and deferred wages in union activity. Although in practice pensions are paid out of the contributions of the current workforce, the productivity of that workforce is itself determined by the investment of labour time of previous workers. Those who see the historical dynamism of capitalism as transforming the modern world tend to see older people as historically irrelevant and as part of the exploiters rather than the exploited.

The concept of exploitation, which lies at the core of many theories of class, provides a material basis to underpin an analysis of social inequality. Exploitation can be conceived of as a lack of balance between the productive labour put into society and the reward, in terms of the available benefits people are able to experience from that collective labour. The idea of labour time measures how much time and effort people contribute to the social endeavour which is society. However, there are significant differences between how much labour time some people put into the social enterprise and how much they take out in terms of both consumption and accumulated assets. Surplus value is the difference in terms of labour time between that which contributes to the total of society's production and that which is received in return.

The flows of surplus value around society are extremely complex. How surplus value is distributed to different sections of society is subject to conflict, manipulation and disguise. These patterns of exploitation are many and varied. The ways in which such surplus value comes to be acquired, controlled and used by groups, institutions or individuals are not always immediately obvious as instances of exploitation. Further, the forms in which labour time is realized as material objects such as aeroplanes or castles, or less tangible things such as power, or leisure or yet other valued things, are equally complex. The ways in which such surplus value is produced, how it is distributed around society and who consumes what part of society's total productivity is a function of the social structure of that society. Exploitation is the systematic accumulation of surplus value by one section of the population that has been produced by another. Exploitation and thus class interests are built up from complex social structures and include not just the institutions of production but consumption and distribution as well. I use the terms production, distribution and consumption as in the standard functional classification of economic activity. This is to avoid the convoluted semantics that have led some writers to say that consumption can sometimes be production in order to preserve the Marxist orthodoxy that exploitation can only occur through production.

Erik Olin Wright (1985) has demonstrated the complexity of class relationships in modern capitalism with the possibilities of being both exploiter and exploited at the same time. He uses the term "ambiguous class locations" to indicate that there is not a simple division of society into two groups, the exploiters and the exploited, and yet retains the central idea that there is a necessary imbalance between effort and reward in capitalist society. It is possible to make an analogous point, that the balance between being exploiter or exploited varies at different points in a life course. The ambiguity Wright refers to becomes even more salient when applied to life courses and not merely occupationally defined "class locations". Thus exploitation and class relationships should not be seen in terms of a constricted view of production and thus limited to a narrowly defined industrial proletariat. It is essential to abandon the idea that production narrowly or simply defined is the sole locus of exploitation. Many aspects of distribution and even consumption must also be looked at as part of the process of creating utility in society (Mingione 1981, Redclift & Mingione 1985, Hamnett 1989) and as having the potential for generating exploitative relationships. Various recent debates have focused on how to understand aspects of this complexity. An understanding of the relationship between inequality and old age requires further questions to be asked about production, distribution and consumption of surplus value. It would therefore seem sensible, in analytic terms, to look at the complexity of social life and identify a variety of processes through which people can be both "exploiters" and "exploited" at the same time, and in particular how the balance between the two can vary over a life-time. Further, it is necessary to look at activities that have been described as distribution and consumption to disentangle the total complex of relationships which enables more powerful groups to gain access to surplus value in society at the expense of the weaker. The material basis of the power of some consumer and commercial interests and the weakness of others, including elderly people, can then be more clearly understood.

Unequal and "exploitative" access to the surplus value generated by social activity can be obtained and denied through a wide range of production, distribution and consumption activities. Domestic production that does not involve wage labour, and in which the categories production, distribution and consumption may be blurred, can lead to exploitation. How women's unpaid labour as mothers and housewives contributes to the cheap production of new workers has been widely discussed and outlined in an earlier section of this chapter. Such arguments have been less well rehearsed with respect to the contribution of the elderly generation to production; a contribution that includes not only support in raising children and servicing those in the workforce with domestic support, but also in the unpaid domestic work of the caring for elderly disabled people who would otherwise require the paid labour of professional carers. Exploitation of unpaid domestic labour is a relatively conventional approach to the idea of exploitation. This view would see retired people, in the same way as housewives, as part of the reproduction of labour power; that is as a mechanism for confining some essential work, which would otherwise fall as a cost to the capitalist production system, to the domestic sphere. Workers require a minimum income level to sustain themselves over the entire course of their lives. Only when they have other alternatives, like returning to the *shamba* (African homestead) or the peasant smallholding and household in old age, can capitalism (short of compulsory euthanasia) avoid the cost of subsistence for the elderly. Exploitation occurs because non-commodified household labour sustains the ability of a section of the household to perform productive labour for the owners of capital in return for less than its full value. In the context of the family, just as housework is not a commodity that is paid for, similarly being old and sustaining the elderly, is non-commodifiable. The contradictions between family and capitalist labour are revealed by the resistance

114

that there is to "caring" for profit (Phillips et al. 1988). Those who care for elderly people are mostly the elderly themselves (Arber & Ginn 1990); they provide valued services for others in the community and when their husbands and wives and their brothers and sisters need support they are the most likely to provide it (Arber & Gilbert 1989, Qureshi & Walker 1989, Ungerson 1987). But because such support is unpaid, it does not enter national incomes calculations or the purview of those attempting to measure intergenerational flows of wealth and income.

It may be that capitalism can survive without exploiting workers through their wages, if it can recoup its surplus value in other ways from those workers when they have retired. There are exploitative relationships that are based on the institutions of consumption. These adversely affect elderly people in so far as they are vulnerable or exploitable consumers. Questions about the power of consumers of different kinds will also give insights into patterns of exploitation in our society. Consumption patterns are structured through forms of control, for example by state monopolies and the marketing policies of large corporations, as well as being manipulated through the media and other cultural institutions. Consumption is part of the systematic structuring of inequality in late modern society. Urban studies have been particularly concerned with inequalities associated with consumption patterns. Mingione's (1981) discussion of the place of consumption in our systems of social reproduction is constructed in an attempt to understand patterns of urban poverty. In Britain the salience of housing and the private ownership of housing has led to a debate on the creation of consumption cleavages in contemporary society. Saunders (1981) has pointed to the differences between those dependent on collective consumption for such things as housing, health and education, and those that are able to use privatized consumption. This approach sees the decomposition of class politics in the 1980s as associated with such consumption cleavages and points to the development of an underclass dependent on poor quality and unreliable collective consumption. The argument I am advancing here is somewhat different but is based on the broader insight into the complexity of the distribution of social value and thus inequality. Saunders (1981) uses the analytic distinction between production and consumption, but puts most emphasis on public versus private consumption. In this part of the argument my central point is that exploitation, conceived in a suitably broad manner, is the concept that can transcend the production/consumption distinction, so that overpricing by public or private organizations and payment of exploitative wage rates can both be seen to have similar effects. Both mechanisms channel surplus value in the interests of capital. The social and political fragmentation that stems from multiple consumption cleavages has a converse in the common sentiments generated by the joint experience of large numbers of people in facing exploitative control from those who supply goods and services to society. The wave of opposition to the imposition of Value Added Tax on fuel and resentment at privatized water charges are an example of these consumer sentiments articulated politically.

A more innovative perspective on the exploitation of the elderly would be to follow those who have challenged the orthodox view that exploitation can only occur within the production process. It is true by definition that only labour power creates value, because it is only by work that natural things can be transformed into useful ones. The real issue is, however, who gains the benefit from that work. In the jargon of this kind of sociology the key question is: What is the method by which surplus value is realized in the circuit of capital from commodity to commodity? The classic equation in which Marx identifies the sources of the extraction of surplus value assumes the existence of a free market; a free market for labour, but most importantly a free market in the supply of goods to the consumer. Thus classically the realization of surplus value for the capitalist entrepreneur is seen as coming from the non-payment for labour time supplied by his workforce. However, in the absence of a proper free market (a condition that empirically must be very rare), monopolistic tendencies may enable capitalists to extract surplus value not from their workers but their consumers. Expressed on a very simplistic level people can be exploited not merely in their role as workers but also in their role as consumers. The capitalist system could continue to work even if workers were paid fully for their labour by their employers as long as a degree of monopoly power enabled surplus value to be accumulated by the over-charging consumers. Many people are both workers and consumers, but many are only consumers; the bourgeois as a class can exploit them by over-charging them for goods they are compelled to purchase. If the collective power of consumers is less than the collective power of workers then the logical strategy for a capitalist class is to increase prices rather than lower wages. Certain groups outside organized wage labour, or in secondary labour markets, such as minorities, women and the elderly, would of course be highly disadvantaged by such a system. Much of the modern world economy is dominated by enormous enterprises, whose power to restrict levels of competition is such, that it is not surprising that many people's subjective sense of exploitation comes from the prices they have to pay as much as from the wages they receive.

Why is this form of exploitation more likely to affect the elderly than other groups in society? Life-course situation structures vulnerability to such exploitation. Elderly people are likely merely to be consumers. Having completed their working lives as employees they cannot seek to share the capitalist's excess profits through wage bargaining but are victims of overpricing. At the end of their life course, elderly people are likely to be consuming a higher proportion of their income than younger age groups by, for example, running down rather than accumulating savings. Because of life-course characteristics, elderly people tend to have small households, and are therefore small-scale and relatively powerless consumers. In so far as terms of trade benefit bulk purchasers, elderly people as small-scale and relatively poor consumers are less likely to carry bargaining power. Elderly people are less mobile, less able to shop around and let the market work in their favour. This inability to use the market also reflects *The poor pay more* work on poverty (Caplovitz 1963), which demonstrates how consumer prices and credit are more expensive for the inner city poor. These effects are seen most clearly in the pricing structure for basic utilities like gas, electricity and water. The standing charge is greatly resented by elderly people as small consumers faced with a disproportionately high price, relative to their consumption, for vital commodities that are essential to daily life.

The argument is then that there is a redistribution away from elderly people in our society mediated through the pricing policies of monopoly or monopsony suppliers. In particular the surpluses of state and newly privatized public utilities are bolstered by standing charges and exploitative prices that fall disproportionately on certain groups including the elderly. Rigidity in the stratification system is facilitated by the fact that those with large amounts of capital can invest securely in, for example, government stocks or public utilities. Transfers of resources are channelled through public sector borrowing and state-determined prices and charges. The elderly person's fixed charge to gain access to monopoly-supplied gas heating ends up in the accumulated capital of those who control the financial markets. It may be that many wealthy elderly people have been able to benefit from these processes of capital accumulation. My argument is that this condition of exploitation through prices will tend to affect old people as a whole because of their small households; their patterns of consumption; their particular structure of needs in housing and heating; and their patterns of income. Thus old age pensioners are apparently powerless in the face of monopolistic pressures that force up their costs as consumers. They were able to bargain collectively as workers when employed but once retired this bargaining counter disappears and they are only left with their voice as citizens of the state to attempt to redress their exploitation. Real unalienated choice is created by proper pensions and also fair prices.

Exploitation is patterned geographically; people in different places experience structured variation in their access to the fruits of social production. How do the patterns of distribution in our society both geographically and socially affect the elderly? There are unequal relationships of distribution in modern society that can adversely affect elderly people in a number of ways. Clearly the lack of access to key institutions such as hypermarkets, the motorway network, efficient public transport or the stock market affect the power of elderly people to command a share of social production. Elderly people's access to the means of distribution is limited by, for example, physical disability, available forms of transport and social barriers of poverty and ageism.

Life-course perspective on exploitation

How does elderly people's access to the good things in life reflect that which they have contributed to society through the course of their lives? Understanding the disadvantaged position of elderly people we need to look at a history of exploitation across the life course. Their access to the fruits of social production is limited by the power structures of advanced capitalism including the patterns of production, distribution and consumption. These problems are of course not unique to elderly people, but the age-based distribution of income and levels of living, for both elderly and young, and issues of race and gender can all be understood in these terms. The use of the concept of the life course can avoid the unreal atomization that compartmentalizes people into productive and unproductive; it rather sees people's lives as embedded in a complex series of unequal overlapping economic relationships.

The way communities and regions are linked to each other in hierarchies of exploitative relationships has been examined from a number of perspectives (Corbridge 1986), for example Wallerstein (1979) has developed his world-system theory. Other theories of underdevelopment, such as those which derive from the work of Arghiri Emmanuel (1972) on unequal exchange, point out how surplus value is distributed around a global system of inequality. Other dependency writers stress the linked hierarchies of exploitation whereby some metropoles are satellites to yet other centres of extraction (Frank 1967). The point is to understand the analogous "geography" of social relationships that locates class, race, gender, age and other systematic inequalities on the "social map".

It is possible to develop an analogy between the world-system theory approach to underdevelopment and the analysis of the position of the elderly in modern capitalism. These approaches have included attempts to comprehend global inequalities of gender, race and class in the advanced capitalist economies (Wallerstein 1974, 1979; Smith et al. 1984). One powerful insight of this school has been to demonstrate the development of underdevelopment, that areas that appear to be backward, poor and underdeveloped now are not simply traditional relics but areas highly exploited in the past. By analogy, the elderly in our society may be viewed as a parallel to those areas, like the villages of Cornish tin miners, Amazonian rubber boom towns, or the ex-steel towns of northern Britain, which have been left as decaying reminders of past economic dynamism. These places, with old people left behind living in the wasted industrial muscle of the past, are the geographical expression equivalent to the burnt-out, retired worker. However, this image has its limitations in a theoretical weakness of the formulation of dependency theory. It is sometimes unclear in such writing whether the poor of the Third World are poor because they are too firmly integrated into world capitalism and thus become highly exploited; or whether they are only marginally attached to the world economy and thus poor because they are not exploited enough. Are elderly people poor because they were exploited in the past, or are they poor because they are currently marginal to the central productive process? The

119

answer is probably both; over the course of a life-time they are exploited in a wide variety of ways and thus the two perspectives may not be incompatible.

Valuing the skills of elder women

The way in which contemporary society constructs images of consumers, concentrating on the young and excluding the old (Friedan 1993), can be linked to the basic need of capitalist economies to grow. The constant need to find new sources of profit leads to both expanded consumption and recruitment of exploitable workers. The marginalization of women and the elderly to insecure and low-paid sections of the labour market makes them more exploitable. Capitalism's need to raise the status of big spending consumers reduces older women, in contrast, to being seen as unwanted and undesirable. It must culturally construct consumers in an image that overvalues conspicuous material consumption (Packard 1963, Redclift 1984) and culturally undervalues the activity of those it wishes to exploit. However, these same attributes are undermining advanced industrial capitalism. The alienation – meaningless work, manipulated consumption, commercialized social relationships – endemic in such societies creates a profound unease. Older women are the victims of the modern consumer capitalism; in many cases those who are most victimized by a social system hold the key to its replacement.

The drive to consumerism creates problems for the environment as well as people. There is a growing awareness that the crisis of capitalism manifests itself as crises of the environment. Raw material shortage, finite supply of oil was in the forefront of environmental consciousness in the 1970s because of the dramatic oil price rises. These problems remain but other crises have also been revealed. Pollution from industrial processes not only lead to direct poisoning but also to insidious changes in the ecological balance. Destruction of the ozone layer, the health risks that result, and the changes in gaseous composition of air that result in the greenhouse effect put question marks over current systems of wealth creation. The social consequence of such crises has included concern about the quality of food and a concern to find environmentally friendly production techniques. Where is the knowledge base to find these alternatives? Older women are repositories of skills and knowledge which many regard as obsolete, and which their children until recently have been increasingly reluctant to learn. However, green-minded grandchildren seeking the knowledge of how to make wholesome food from natural products, the skills of domestic production of all types, the most efficient way to recycle household products, and the skills with which to make and mend clothes would do well to ask their grandmothers first. The senior generation of elderly women should be valued for their domestic and craft skills. In particular, rural women have these skills. In places like Britain with long urban traditions of poverty, the "waste not want not" mentality, which is so unfashionable in a consumer society, was essential. Working-class women growing up at the beginning of the century had to have advanced domestic and craft skills. These women have the recycling skills necessary for living lifestyles that are not profligate with the planet's resources. The role of grandmother knowledge in survival may not yet be evolutionally obsolete.

There is a very trenchant criticism of this route to revaluing old people. It romanticizes the hard work and drudgery our grandmothers had to endure. So it is necessary to comment that both men and women need to relearn the skills of living gently on the earth from those women who still remember them. Secondly, while recognizing hard work is not necessarily fun, in the past it was frequently a social occasion. It was both more efficient and more fun to thresh corn, spin or embroider together. Thus the skills cannot be isolated from their social context; environmentally sound techniques of production require their appropriate social relations of production.

Emergent structures

Inequalities have a material base, systematic inequalities are built up by people's actions over time. The increased salience of age-based criteria in the contemporary world is illustrative of this process of emergent structure. By salient I mean that it is likely to be used more frequently by social actors in defining the situation. Through this process old age becomes institutionalized. That is, it becomes a structured part of systematic power relations in societies that constrain and condition people's opportunities and the ways in which they live. However, people do not simply passively receive this institutionalization but think, reevaluate, act and organize around these changes. One way of trying to understand this pattern of "structurization" of age, including the increasing incorporation of age criteria into social power relations, is to compare situations in which age is less salient. For example in small-scale societies, such as rural agriculturally based societies, in which familial institutions are more dominant than the market and in which kinship networks are preferred to formal institutions, age is less salient than in contemporary urban society. It appears to be true of small-scale societies that because they are dealing with people whose histories are known and are viewed as whole (as opposed to partial) social personalities, single categorical criteria are less deterministic than in our large-scale bureaucratized society. The point is not to romanticize face-to-face communities as warmer or more supportive. Intimacy can lead to enmity as well as affection. Rather, I am making the structural point that the social processing of large numbers of people requires simplification of people's public persona, and as a consequence readily available labels such as age become the corner stones of social personality.

A further illustration of the importance of emergent structure lies in the sociology of ethnicity where the analysis of the development of new ethnic groups illustrates emergent structure. The production of social boundaries is an idea that stems from the work of anthropologist Fredrik Barth and which has, for example, stimulated new work in the United States that discusses "racialization" processes, particularly in politics (Barth 1969). This approach sees the development of races not as fixed categories but as new emergent forms – the 1980s have seen the institutionalization of racial definitions and racial forms of action and consciousness in the political sphere in ways that are new but derived from history (Gilroy 1987, Ringer & Lawless 1989). Thus "race" is not the simple reproduction of former racial stereotypes and patterns of racial action but a development of a new politics; an emerging social pattern. Similarly an argument can be made for the historical development and change within the feminist movement. In terms of the reflexive nature of social reproduction, where former structures (for example occupational structures) have been challenged and changed, this leads to new consciousness, new action, new politics, new feminist ways of organizing, which will themselves have further consequences as they are in turn contingently reproduced. Most importantly for this book and the discussion here, it can be argued that in parallel to "racialization" there is an "ageization" (which is such a horrible piece of English I will not use it again). What is meant by this is the process by which the criteria of age come to structure society and relations within it as a self-reinforcing process; the pattern of age inequality is reproduced in stronger form over time by the specific circumstances of contemporary industrial capitalist society. The argument therefore is that in industrial society in the last part of the twentieth century age is becoming much more important in relation to people's experience and is becoming a criterion which more people use to interpret and understand their society and structure their own consciousness and action. Additionally and as a consequence of such increasing salience of age, there are changes in the contingent circumstances of other groups of people, which in turn structures their opportunities and their actions.

Most classical theories of inequality assume that elderly people are of no social significance – they are seen as the residue not the makers of history, or as a functionless element of society shunted to one side as roles pass to successor generations. As Phillipson (1982) remarks, both the productivist emphasis of classical Marxism, which makes male workers the centre of analysis, and Marxist feminists, who make reproduction through domestic labour the central point of debate, implicitly marginalize elderly people. By concentrating on the concept of life course and locating a diversity of life courses within a pattern of global historical change, it should become possible to integrate key elements of theories of gender, race and class into a single approach that represents a major advance in the field of social inequality.

CHAPTER SIX

Numbers and justice:
who's afraid of an ageing population?

The purpose of this chapter is to address the question of whether the demographic changes that have produced an ageing population affect the social position of elderly people *vis-à-vis* other groups in modern Western society. The discussion of inequality and old age can thus be furthered by considering issues of numbers and equity. As can be seen from previous chapters, many of the key debates about the current and future condition of elderly people in modern Western society centre on the functioning and future of the welfare state, and in particular on issues about pensions. Pensions are of essential importance when considering old age inequalities. They are central to the material inequalities of old age; for many people in the industrialized world they are the sole means of keeping body and soul together. Culturally they are significant in establishing social definitions of old age and the process by which people internalize a sense of being old. The question of pensions is becoming increasingly sensitive as numbers of academics and politicians query the possibility of sustaining, let alone improving, levels of pensions provision in the face of demographic change and an ageing population (Smeeding 1991). In the final part of this chapter, I will consider if the current debates on the future of pensions' systems constitute a threat to the status of elderly people.

The demography of ageing populations

It is necessary to discuss the numbers of elderly people and the changing patterns of population in order to establish the nature of the demographic issues and place them in due proportion. Although it is appropriate to start with these demographic considerations, it should not be taken for granted that increasing numbers of elderly people necessarily constitute a problem. Social problems do not exist independently of power relations. Social issues are the problems defined by particular sections of society and arise from particular social relationships and interests. They are not intrinsic to any demographic pattern *per se*.

How many old people are there in Britain and what proportion of the population do they represent? According to the 1991 census there were 11,461,906 people of 60 years or over in Great Britain – 3,853,569 were 75 or more years old – out of a total of 54,156,068. The 1991 census (OPCS 1993b) reports that pensioners (assumed to

Table 6.1 Population of Great Britain, males 65 and over and females 60 and over, 1851–1991.

Year	Total population (millions)	Older people (millions)	Proportion of elderly (%)	Average annual increase (%)
1851	20.8	1.3	6.1	
1861	23.1	1.4	6.2	1.2
1871	26.1	1.6	6.1	1.1
1881	29.7	1.8	6.1	1.4
1891	33.0	2.1	6.2	1.2
1901	37.0	2.3	6.2	1.1
1911	40.8	2.7	6.7	1.9
1921	42.8	3.3	7.8	2.0
1931	44.8	4.3	9.6	2.5
1941	–	–	–	–
1951	48.8	6.7	13.6	2.2
1961	51.3	7.6	14.7	1.3
1971	54.0	8.7	16.2	1.5
1981	54.3	9.6	17.7	0.9
1991	54.1	10.4	18.7	0.8

Source: Warnes 1987: 42, modified by the author using the 1991 census; see also Thane 1989: 59.

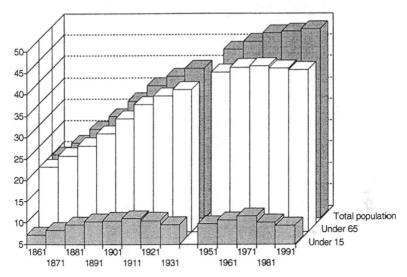

Figure 6.1 Total population by age group, England and Wales 1861–1991. *Source:* author's analysis of OPCS 1993a.

...e women of 60 and over, men of 65 and over) form 18.7% of the Great Britain population, this is an 0.8% increase in the ten years since 1981. The proportion of people who are 75 years and over has increased 0.5% for men and 0.8% for women, between the 1981 census and the 1991 census. Of all British households 33.5% have at least one pensioner whereas 24.8% of British households consist only of pensioners.

Table 6.1 details the change in the British population of pensionable age over a 140-year period. It shows the numbers of such people, the percentage of the total population they represent, and in the final column an indication of the speed at which the proportion of elderly people in the population is increasing (this is calculated by taking the increase in the numbers of pensionable age from one census to the next, expressing this as a percentage of the former, and dividing by ten to obtain an annual rate).

In 1851 when the population was recorded as 20.8 million there were only 1.3 million of "pensionable age" (6.1% of the population). The percentage of elderly people in the population remained static at around 6.2% until the census of 1911, by which time the population of the country as a whole had doubled to 40.8 million. It was around

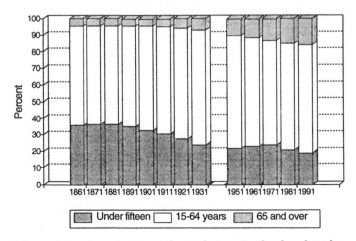

Figure 6.2 Age structure of population, England and Wales 1861–1991. *Source:* author's analysis of OPCS 1993a.

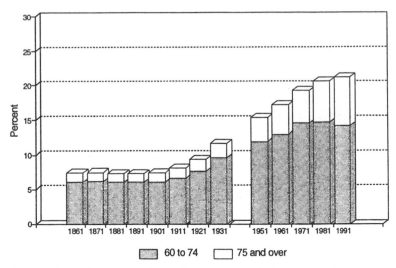

Figure 6.3 Age composition of elderly population, England and Wales 1861–1991. *Source:* author's analysis of OPCS 1993a.

this time that the proportion of the population in the pensionable age range started to grow significantly. The annual increase in the population counted as elderly grew from 1.1% to nearly 2%. The acceleration in the numbers of pensionable-age people in the British population reached its peak in the 1931 census at which time the population was 44.8 million of whom 4.3 million were of pensionable age (9.6% of the population). The number of pensioners in the population was at this time increasing by 2.5% per annum, subsequently this rate of growth declined. Although the absolute numbers of pensioners continued to grow, this happened at a less fast rate. In the 1981 census there were 54.3 million people in Great Britain, 9.6 million of whom where of pensionable age and this represented 17.7% of the population as a whole. However, the average annual increase in numbers of pensioners had declined to less than one per cent. The way in which these trends changed the size of the population of different ages in England and Wales over a similar period can be seen from Figure 6.1. Figure 6.2 illustrates the changing proportions of young and old people in the population.

The proportion of over 75-year-olds in England and Wales is undergoing change at an even more accelerated rate than that for those of pensionable age. This is illustrated in Figure 6.3. An important transition was experienced in population structure recorded in the 1971 census, whereby the declining fertility rates sixty to seventy years ago expressed themselves as a stabilizing in the trend of an ageing population. However, the proportion of the very elderly (those over 75) in British society will continue to rise. This pattern of growth in the very elderly population can be illustrated by OPCS population projections based on the results of the 1991 census (see Table 6.2). In their estimation, the total population will grow by 7.8%, from 57.6 million in 1991 to 62.1 million by the year 2031. By 2011 the percentage of those over retirement age will have increased from 18.4% to 19.5%, but the numbers of over retirement age projected for 2031 will have grown by 51.8%. Between 1991 and 2031 the numbers over 75 years in age are projected to grow by 70% (OPCS 1993e).

Table 6.2 Projected population in millions, United Kingdom 1991–2031.

	1991	2001	2011	2021	2031
Children under 16	11.7	12.5	11.9	11.5	11.4
Men 65–74 and women 60–74	6.6	6.3	7.3	8.4	9.3
All 75 and over	4.0	4.5	4.7	5.5	6.8
All ages	57.6	59.7	61.1	62.0	62.1

Source: OPCS 1993e.

Mortality

People have to die of something. Historically in the Western world there has been a changing pattern in the causes of death. The infectious diseases and the diseases of childhood, by themselves or exacerbated by the effects of malnutrition, are no longer the killers they were in the past. In modern Western Europe the major killers are the chronic diseases, particularly cardiovascular problems and cancer. Further, accident and suicide are, over large parts of the life span, the most frequent cause of death. The major causes of increases in people's longevity over the last one hundred and fifty years have been summarized as peace, potatoes and penicillin (Goldthorpe 1975: 24, quoting Myrdal 1945: 17). Better public health measures, including safe water and sanitation along with immunization, have been the major medical contribution to an increased life span. Thus penicillin in the quote stands for antibiotics, and also vaccination and other public health measures, which have enabled increasing proportions of people in the West to avoid the killer infections of the past. Economic growth, particularly the expansion of world food supplies and the growth both in productivity and international trade in food, has meant that many people are less susceptible to famine and malnutrition, and the diseases associated with them. Thus the potatoes in the quote stand for the increased food production available following the distribution of New World crops such as maize and potatoes to the other continents of the world. Peace is a problematic idea, as over the course of history warfare has been increasingly industrialized and exported; the potential for death from the activities of hostile strangers has greatly increased, but members of Western society are less likely to die at the hands of one of their own nation than at many times in the past. Technical innovation has also increased the chance of mass accidental mortality; there are increased chances of death ranging from car accidents to accidental nuclear emissions. The achievement of a sufficient level of world peace to enable regular, large-scale trade in basic commodities, such as food and fertilizer, is probably the most significant contribution "peace" has made to longevity.

Life expectancy

Although life expectancy is increasing, there is no evidence of an increase in absolute achievable longevity. This is because by far the largest decline in death has been in the area of infant mortality and life expectancy statistics are conventionally reported as life expectancy at birth. The chances of mothers surviving pregnancy have also greatly increased over this century. This has had the effect of concentrating the age of death in the 70- and 80-year-old age group. Some writers have called this the rectangular survival curve. Greatly increased life expectancy at birth over the last hundred and fifty years is not reflected in a similarly large increase in life expectancy at age 70 or 80. Changes in longevity have been largely associated with changing social conditions. The role of medical science in elongating the basic biological life span is debatable. The media frequently report apparent breakthroughs in medical science that will produce longevity. However, the discussion in Chapter 4 of the place of medical science in our current cultural construction of old age might explain the continued search and optimistic reporting of quasi immortality. On the other hand, there is evidence of a social expectation of the age of death and medical teams striving with less than total determination to preserve the life of the very old who have reached such an age (Sudnow 1967).

In the last twenty years in Britain there has been some increase in life expectancy at birth, although it is not large when compared to the previous sixty (*Social Trends* 1994). Indeed for some sections of the population, particularly young lower-class men, mortality rates during the 1980s have actually shown an increase. It is not the contribution of hospitals, surgery and "heroic" medicine that has changed the average length of the life span. It is very mundane preventative measures informed by medical science that have made the difference. The groups in the USA that have exhibited the greatest increase in life expectancy in recent years have been those groups most at risk of coronary heart disease but who have changed diet and lifestyles. Britain has been somewhat slow in following these trends (Joshi 1989: 7).

Global demographic changes

The distribution of elderly people in the world relates to issues of development. The demographic transition model is frequently the basis for discussion of population issues and economic development. Key points of this model are that development leads to a decline in the death rate that is subsequently followed some years later by a decline in the birth rate. In the context of ageing populations, this model suggests that the rate of the ageing is affected strongly by the rate of decline in the propensity of women to have babies. The model also predicts an expanded but stable proportion of elderly people in the population, once the effects of the lower birth and death rates have worked themselves through (see Table 6.3). It is important to note that in future the most rapidly ageing populations will be in the Third World where the decline in the fertility rate has been most rapid. The largest gains in life expectancy in recent years have also been made in the Third World which will further increase the absolute numbers of elderly people (Sen 1994).

The speed at which people change their fertility-regulating behaviour and therefore have fewer children affects the rate of ageing of the population. These demographic patterns are repeated in both developed and underdeveloped countries. Although of course varying in

Table 6.3 Number of people aged 65 or over, international comparisons (in millions).

	1950	1975	2000	2025
China	24.9	40.8	90.4	193.9
India	12.0	23.7	81.3	118.9
USA	12.4	22.7	34.0	59.6
USSR (former)	10.4	23.4	33.6	48.5
Japan	4.1	8.8	20.7	31.0
Indonesia	3.2	4.3	11.0	25.9
Brazil	1.3	4.0	9.7	22.8
Pakistan	2.1	2.2	4.7	13.3
Mexico	1.1	2.1	4.7	11.6
Bangladesh	1.5	2.8	4.9	10.8
Nigeria	0.8	1.6	4.0	9.9

Source: calculated from United Nations 1993; (cf. Alex Kalache "Ageing and developing countries: a new challenge", British Society of Gerontology Conference 20–22 September 1991, quoted in Johnson & Falkingham 1992: 47).

specific detail, the ageing of the population is visible or predictable across most of the world, Japan being the country with the most dramatic and extreme pattern of ageing. In 1960, Japan had a situation of 9 people aged 65 and over for every 100 aged 15–64 (this is a standard formula used to calculate the so-called "dependency ratio" of elderly people to the "economically active" population). The comparable figure for the United Kingdom at this time was 17.9 per hundred "economically active" people. However, by 1980 Japan's figure had reached 13.4 and is projected to reach 22.6 by the year 2000 and 32.9 by 2025. Figures for the United Kingdom for the same years are 23.5, 23.3 (in other words, a stable proportion in the last two decades of this century) going up to 29.7 by 2025 (Ermisch 1989: 29). More recent population projections, taking into account the even greater than expected fall in the fertility rate, suggest even higher proportions of elderly people, but the comparative point about the less extreme character of the change in Britain compared to many other countries still remains.

Declining rates of economic participation among elderly people

The assumption is frequently made that the elderly population is economically unproductive. Patterns of work and the reasons for non-participation in the labour market have varied considerably over time, but elderly people have not always withdrawn from work. In Britain in 1881, according to Johnson (1985), 73 per cent of the male population of 65 and over were in employment, but by 1981 the percentage had shrunk to less than 11 per cent. This major change in the distribution of work is not because the population has become physically less able and therefore less employable. Townsend (1986) argues that in the absence of evidence of increased disability among older people, these changing employment patterns must reflect either differing employment practices and/or changing life-course choices by the older population. However, non-employed does not mean non-productive; it may mean productive potential is being lost, or that useful work is not recorded or recognized as such.

There has been a rapid decline in the numbers of older people in work (Guillemard 1989, Laczko & Phillipson 1991). In 1965, 90% of men between 60 and 65 years old were working, but by the end of the 1980s this was down to 60%. Pressures and opportunities for early retirement came with the recession of the early 1980s. Studies also show the number of people on disability benefits varies with the unemployment rate. Doctors apparently take into account the job market when judging "fitness to work"! It is further argued that there has been a breakdown in the traditional pattern of work and retirement; for example, the expectation that people work until 60 or 65 and then retire has changed. There is also much evidence that if employers are willing to recruit older people to work for them there are plenty of elderly people who would like the opportunity. Workers on incremental salary scales close to retirement are relatively expensive and unattractive to new employers, but many employers value the return to work of older employees, who are regarded as reliable and skilled but who are also willing to do less popular, lower-wage or part-time jobs to supplement their pensions. Unfortunately employers also carry many of the ageist stereotypes found in the rest of the population and suspect that illness and inflexibility characterize older workers. The pension debate, and the affordability of social support for the elderly, has to be seen in conjunction with opportunities for meaningful and rewarding work.

Why should the projected shortage of workers not be met by the reversal of this trend with elderly people increasingly participating in the labour force again? The elderly and disabled people in the workforce were forced out during recession, and many of the supposed "retirees" did not perceive their retirement as particularly "voluntary" despite official labels (Guillemard 1989, 1990; Kohli et al. 1992). The excuse for the hardships of unemployment during the slump of the early 1980s was that technological change was displacing labour. Modern automation techniques would provide a world free from want, with everyone gaining more leisure time. Now, a few years later, we are being told that there will be a chronic shortage of labour necessary to sustain us in the standard of living (or at least the levels of pensions) to which we have become accustomed.

Dependency ratios, migration and nationalism

There is a contradiction between the two strands of current British and indeed European population policy. This policy confusion is also reflected on the other side of the Atlantic. On the one hand there is the "apocalyptic demography" which suggests society will be overwhelmed by the needs of elderly people; on the other, there is the fear of being overwhelmed by movements of "economic migrants". These themes stand in contradiction to each other and to the proclaimed ideological basis for current government policy, namely that of the free market. To put the idea of an international free market in labour on the agenda reveals the racist nature of immigration policy, the ageist approach to pensions policy and the essentially reactionary nature of government policies. The identification of elderly people as a problem is designed primarily as a strategy to undermine the role of the state in providing its citizens with pensions and welfare services.

The apocalyptic population projections (Robertson 1991) are based solely on fertility and mortality rates. They fail to take proper account of potential or even foreseeable trends in migration. The construction of the demographic problem is built on the preconceptions that the citizens of the state are those born there and that those contributing to the national pension schemes will be nationals. Neither is true, but both are built around assumptions that citizenship of the state is based on descent and race rather than political rights and duties. This attitude reflects a nationalism that equates the nation with a genetically based group recruited by biological reproduction, rather than for example a collection of citizens freely associating themselves with the state (Hobsbawm 1992). Such nationalism also reflects an attitude that sees national culture as homogeneous, monolithic and unchanging, and is unreflectively based on selective historical symbols (Anderson 1991), rather than say pride in current collective progress and achievements. The exclusion of an active consideration of migration in the discussion of these demographic issues is to make the further assumption that immigration is a problem, indeed that it is so self-evidently problematic that it need not figure in the debate.

A further nationalist assumption built into the definition of the problem is that the national economy coincides with the borders of the state, either in geographical terms or in terms of citizenship. Numbers of countries have a significant part, even a majority, of their working population who are non-citizens. Conversely, some countries have a majority of their working population working abroad, and in some cases contributing to the pension schemes of the host countries. The major economic institutions of the world are multinational in character, be they multinational firms such as Ford or Philips, or supra-national institutions such as the EC or the World Bank. Neither the contributions, nor the investments or the payments from a pension scheme are limited to the boundaries of the state. In terms of funded schemes, even at present significant portions of British pension funds are invested abroad, and accumulate value through the work of overseas labour. We live in a global economy and a global society and, therefore, to consider these demographic issues on the basis of individual or small groups of countries in isolation is to manufacture an artificial problem.

If we set aside these narrowly focused and nationalist assumptions and look at the global situation, we find that the world population profile in 1975 was younger than it has ever been. Although there has been some change since then, particularly in Third World fertility, in gross terms, one-third of the population of the world is still under 15 (Valkovics 1989: table 4). What is more, a significant number of young people are not only keen but desperate for the opportunity to work in the industrialized economies. All major industrialized countries have severe restrictions on immigration. Ever more elaborate procedures are being implemented to stem the tide of people seeking new opportunities in the very countries identified as having a "problem" of ageing. Indeed such is the concern of European governments to exclude economic migration, that they are changing the human rights legislation that guarantees refugees the right of asylum. So-called economic migrants are sifted from the growing numbers of asylum seekers arriving at the borders of the West, and degrading scenes on the borders of the industrialized world see not only Vietnamese forcibly deported from Hong Kong, Sri Lankan Tamils imprisoned without trial in Britain, Romanian gypsies entering Germany sent back as unacceptable, but innumerable similar occurrences repeated daily. If our demography leaves us short of workers and the changing dependency ratio is a problem, why are we keeping these people out? It is only when viewed from a narrowly nationalistic basis that there can be concerns about changing dependency ratios. There are plenty of young people across the world ready and willing to work (and be trained) in the economies of those countries with large numbers of elderly people. It is therefore clear that the real issue is not demographic and the hidden agenda is nationalism. There is no relationship between the size of population groups and how well off they are. Satisfactory material lifestyles for elderly people depend on productivity and economic growth and the distribution of the wealth generated by such growth.

It is bizarre that no-one seems to put these issues of population policy together. An ageing population and immigration of young workers are simultaneously seen as problems. Even more extraordinary is that this blindness should come from the monetarist right governments that dominate the industrialized world. Those, who for more than a decade have been not only advocating the virtues of the market but also implementing market models in public services and privatizing anything with a sale value, nevertheless seem blind to the virtues of a free market in labour. The Conservatives in Britain freed capital and currency from exchange controls almost as one of the first acts of the 1979 Thatcher administration. The right in Britain has continually advocated the virtues of free trade and opposed import controls. Yet perversely they have increased restrictions on the mobility of labour.

A freer world market in labour could well provide the economic impetus necessary to shift the world out of recession, which increasing economic nationalism can merely exacerbate. Not only would such a policy create an expanding global market in consumer products, but it would also provide a ready way around the inflationary labour bottlenecks of an expanding economy. There is a strong historical association between immigration in Europe and economic growth. It has usually been assumed, without much analysis, that economic growth was the cause of the immigration effect in postwar Europe. However, it is plausible that cause and effect were the other way around; that the freer market for labour and thus greater labour migration (or at least the absence of draconian restrictions) led to growth in the economy.

How might the welfare state affect inequality and the status of elderly people?

Those who see inequality as a feature of social structure and manifest in the material circumstances of different sections of society look to the creation of new institutions to redress this inequality. In particular, reformers have looked to the state to provide that role, and in Western Europe the specific form of the welfare state has developed. Understanding the material inequalities experienced by elderly people in Western society depends on grasping how the welfare state affects their interests. However, it remains a matter of dispute as to whether the welfare state does redistribute wealth to the needy and create increased social equality, or whether it maintains the interests of dominant groups and so preserves inequality. Is the welfare state a class-based phenomenon, or is it a feature of industrial society and independent of political ideology? Are elderly people the victims of the welfare state, which has sapped their independence and created an age-based underclass dependent on state benefits? Alternatively, the welfare state might be seen as the triumph of collective provision, which enables the benefits of economic growth to be spread in a civilized manner to all members of society, including those who have retired. Conversely, what impact do elderly people have on the welfare state? Is welfare spending a function of economic interests, and consequent upon the size and power of groups like the elderly? Do the increased numbers of pensioners in advanced industrial democracies give elderly people political clout to obtain welfare expenditures in disproportionate amounts, or is it unlikely that the elderly form an effective interest group?

Marshall (1950) suggested that modern political systems have advanced, first by the people achieving political rights, then civil rights and subsequently welfare rights – roughly coinciding with progress from the eighteenth, to the nineteenth and to the twentieth centuries. Views as to the motor for these social changes differ. There are those who see this progress achieved by struggles that have wrestled these rights from the power of the privileged. However, there are those who see such change progressing from the logic of the efficient functioning of modern society. Those taking the latter point of view are more likely to advocate equality of opportunity, emphasizing not only its moral appeal, but also its efficient use of talents. However, this is not the fundamental meaning of equality; laws that might give all at birth an equal million to one chance to hold monopoly of power, wealth and privilege would not reduce inequality. It is of no consolation to the slave that a few slaves may escape and join the ranks of the slave owners. The liberal idea of individualistic equality, linked to equality before the law and the absence of feudal or inherited privilege, needs to be combined with the socialist recognition of the collective nature of social production and therefore the rights of the collectivity to share in the benefits of that production. Tawney (1931) like many others believed that the welfare state could achieve this.

Nowadays there is less confidence in the role of the state, and there are radically differing views as to who gains and who loses by the advance of the welfare state. It is even unclear as to who are the key powerful players in the drama. Pampel & Williamson (1989) suggest there are four principal approaches to these questions about the nature and function of the welfare state; industrialism theory, monopoly capitalism theory, social democratic theory and interest group theory. Industrialism theory suggests that the welfare state developed to meet the needs of modern industrial society; it serves to provide a healthy, educated, flexible labour supply, with socially acceptable ways of supporting those not directly in employment. This kind of approach undervalues the history of political struggles that led to the creation of modern welfare institutions. Health and welfare benefits for the elderly have been hotly contested issues and a functionally efficient meritocracy is not a Utopia that solves the problem of inequality. The monopoly capitalism approach sees the welfare state and the pension as a device of dominant groups in society to keep the working class pacified. Dependent people then have an interest in the little security that the status quo provides them, and are unlikely therefore to support radical change; the first state pension schemes were introduced in Germany by a conservative regime deliberately setting out to steal the thunder of the left (Kohli 1991). Although the way in which right-dominated governments in the 1980s have been assiduously undermining the welfare state in the name of the free market does not suggest they see things in this way.

Interest group theory reflects the American experience and sees welfare provision in society as a function of political pluralism whereby a variety of interest groups contend, through the political arena, for a share of society's benefits. Social democratic theory identifies the welfare state as part of a historic compromise between capital and labour. From this perspective pensions and the welfare state are particular achievements of the west European labour and social democratic movements, that have succeeded in modifying capitalism to incorporate welfare ends. Clearly the structure of politics and the distribution of political power are the key to understanding the development of pensions and welfare provision for the elderly.

Power structures give force to inequality in terms of the material conditions of people's lives. The intentions of egalitarian welfare legislation may be undermined by powerful groups in society. The social context in which a social policy is developed may have more to do with the positive or negative consequences for inequality than with the terms of the policy itself. Further, the meaning of inequality derives from a historical context, so that how people interpret social change will vary. Therefore, understanding the significance of changes in pensions and welfare policies cannot be done in abstract but needs to be related to specific times and places.

The discussions of generational equity which have been particularly powerful in the United States have focused on whether, rather than elderly people being a disadvantaged sector of the population, they are consuming more than their fair share of society's resources to the detriment of younger groups, particularly children. Contrary to the argument that there is a problem of age inequality which all experience in later life in modern societies, numbers of writers have sought to identify the up-coming generation of elderly people as privileged compared to future generations.

As we have seen, the apocalyptic demographers and the new right financiers are looking for ways in which to convince people that current pension arrangements are unsustainable. Their view ignores the fact that population ageing has been going on for some time and that we are not demographically in a new situation (Laczko & Phillipson 1991: 107). The preceding demographic discussion shows that the rate of ageing of the British population was at its highest at precisely the time during which the British pension system was being established. The average age of the British population started to increase in the first decade of the twentieth century, the rate of increase in the proportion of people over retirement age peaked in the 1930s and the proportion of people over retirement age in the last decade of this century is unlikely to increase at all. Nevertheless, at the time when its population was ageing most rapidly, the British pension system was established and expanded, and proved very popular even though the working population was being expected to find larger and larger sums to support these schemes. This historical precedent would suggest that over an 80-year period we could see a 15 per cent increase in the proportion of our population over retirement age and a substantial increase in the value of the pension, provided of course that the economic growth equivalent to that same period was repeated.

Is there a problem of generational equity? Those writing within the "life-course perspective" have raised this challenge (Johnson 1993). However, a life-course approach can provide answers for these concerns, providing a broad enough view is taken and the sequencing of generations through society is not limited to a minor branch of mathematical logic but is viewed as a key issue in historical sociology. It is important not to limit such debate to abstract models with unrealistic assumptions that are made to enable the optimizing models of economists to be calculated (Cowen & Parfit 1992, Johnson & Falkingham 1992: 149). Taking the issue of the dynamics of funded pension schemes in isolation is a good example where the ignoring of the dimension of the life course, as a historically constructed and culturally meaningful process, can distort our perception of elderly people.

Particularly in America, but also in Europe and the Antipodes, there has been a fierce debate both in the academic and popular press about the issue of generation equity. It has focused most strongly on the extent to which elders are getting more than their fair share of welfare expenditures at the expense of children (Preston 1984, Moody 1992, Laslett & Fishkin 1992, Johnson 1993). These debates were brought into a British context by Paul Johnson et al. (1989), whose book seeks to provide academic respectability to the monetarist right's attempt to roll back the state by reducing the pension. Careful consideration of the arguments and evidence does not reveal the apocalyptic scenario that Paul Johnson, the principal editor, announced as "increasingly bitter competition for resources between workers and pensioners" (Johnson et al. 1989: 2).

Statements such as "the seeds of the intergenerational conflict are already bearing bitter fruit" and the labelling of the "welfare generation" (which involves the placing of a whole generation in the "scrounger" category) are not borne out either by the presentation of evidence or by the analysis in their book. Without denying there is a political problem in obtaining secure funding for pensions, the time scale and the magnitude of the necessary changes do not seem to me to require the gloomy attitudes to pensioners' rights that have been adopted (Walker 1990a).

Paul Johnson et al.'s (1989) argument is based around the idea of a "generational contract" that is closely related to Moody's (1992) "generational compact" and other works within the American tradition of writing on the ethics of old age (Laslett 1992). The uncritical application of the idea of a social contract to the relationships between generations is a weakness in much of the discussion of generational equity. The concept of a generational contract is developed entirely as a philosophical tool with which to hypothesize about alternative moral positions. It is important not to confuse stories told in mythical mode about original or primordial relationships in order to make a moral point with attempts at empirically based historical description. Questions such as "How do generations enter contracts? What decision-making mechanism exists for entering such a contract?" cannot be answered because they would require historical data. However, in practice even the metaphorical use of the contract analogy tends to be restricted to moral speculation without sufficient close reference to the idea of a social contract within political theory. Rousseau (1762) based his theory of social order on the concept of consenting individuals and saw his social contract as one made among the citizens of society. His mythical story was used to explain what should be understood as the morality of government.

There are of course many other theories of the state and the nature of social cohesion that do not resort to the idea of the social contract and that are equally applicable to the nature of the integration of pensioners into contemporary society. The political economy approach is one such analysis that I will develop in the following chapter. The idea of a contract involves a variety of assumptions – individual consent, freely given, on the basis of knowledge and understanding, and *equally* binding on the contracting parties. There are clearly other models of possible or desirable social relationships. There is no need to take recourse to such conceptual devices as a generational contract to study the reciprocal relationship of pensioners to the rest of society. Further issues of moral responsibility between generations, even those who are historically separate and include the as yet unborn, are very real. Discourse that reduces morality to the image of bargainers in a market is not necessary, and indeed is inadequate, when dealing with the mutual responsibilities of human beings to each other particularly when the mankind in question is extended into the future and into the past. The individualism and economism implicit in these discussions of social contracts should be critically examined rather than simply assumed.

The idea of generational equity is the notion that all generations and all age groups have a right to be treated fairly, and that the rights of older people have to be balanced with the competing claims of other age groups. There is some confusion in the debates about equity between age groups, for example children as opposed to people over 70; and equity between cohorts, for example people born in the 1930s as opposed to those born in the 1960s. The context of the debate, however, is the future of the American social security and Medicare systems, and more broadly the role of the state in making transfers through taxation and benefits between generations. In the real world it is difficult to separate chronological age and historical age from one another. Laws and benefits tend to be written in terms of chronological age but benefits and burdens are borne by actual historical individuals and groups.

Most people experience old age not as an abstract category of the demographers or economists but as specific relationships with family, friends and neighbours. Generations are not social categories that readily form groups and articulate interests. Indeed studies give little indication of this kind of political organization in any context other than some recent pressure groups in the United States. In Britain increased organization by pensioners reflects erosion of their pension entitlement but there are no signs of organized opposition from younger age groups. However, people seldom identify with cohort, thus it is difficult for their interests to be expressed or articulated. This inarticulateness is strongest, of course, for the unborn generations. This observation is significant for it is in the name of these unborn generations that important current claims are being made: on the one hand, claims about the environment and not passing the consequences of our pollution and resource depletion to future generations; on the other hand, however, some from the radical right have claimed to champion these future generations from avaricious current cohorts making unsustainable claims to pension provision.

Pensions may be a problem for those politicians trying to cut government expenditure. However, government income and expenditure are political decisions, and are currently based on a specific ideology that takes for granted that expenditure on pensions has lower priority than the defence budget, and that welfare revenues should come from young people's income rather than tax on alcohol consumption. Johnson and others writing on these issues do not adequately address the equity of the current distribution of British national resources. The low proportion of the British national income that is devoted to pensions (7.7% compared to 14.3% in

France or 16.9% in Italy) is unregarded (Walker 1990a: 379). Further, there are issues of future economic productivity. If every British worker was as productive as every German, it is very unlikely that we would have any difficulty in paying substantially increased pensions to the more experienced members of our society.

There is a cross-generational stake in the pension system and the welfare state and this support is consistently shown in surveys of public opinion (Minkler & Cole 1991: 43). People by and large do not identify generations or age groups as in conflict. Younger people support social security and health service (like Medicaid) measures even though they might be pessimistic about those being there in the future for themselves. Why do they take this attitude? Because it "reflects in part the fact that younger people in the workforce prefer to have their parents indirectly supported than to shoulder this burden themselves in a more direct way" (Minkler 1991: 78). However, the moral economy argument is the key to the continued support of younger generations for old age entitlements they believe will go bankrupt before their time. The belief in a moral economy is grounded in a set of values whose central goal is "to structure a society so as to maximise possibilities of a decent life for all" (Hendricks & Leedham 1991: 58).

The irony is that pensioners are more likely to believe that those living on state benefits are less entitled to them than does the general population. It is this set of "scrounger" haters who themselves are being labelled as "scroungers" (Midwinter & Tester 1987). The danger is that if the label sticks, it can be used to cut the living standards of our older fellow citizens. The central moral question contained in the idea of social justice is for many people, both young and old, that they do not want to live in a society where some citizens are living in increasing poverty while others grow rich. This is a communitarian ideal. The problem of equity has less to do with generational justice than common humanity, or more precisely a moral economy – a set of moral precepts that form the basis of social relationships on which an economy must be built. Intergenerational justice does not mean the acceptance of the dangerous new right propositions that equate social justice with fiscal transfers. There has been a failure to consider the issue of the fairness of the social processes that redistribute wealth between the different age groups in society in a broader context than the specific calculus of the mechanisms of the "pay-as-you-go" pension formulae. Such a restricted consideration fails to understand the bonds of interconnectedness within which webs of social obligation are created and feelings of morality and fairness evolve. As a consequence there is a failure to understand the strength of commitment to the welfare state. Indeed there is a danger of a self-fulfilling prophecy developing, whereby if sufficient insecurity and doubt can be spread about the future of the pension, these anxieties will succeed in undermining those webs of social support that currently sustain the pension and leave individuals vulnerable to the whims of the financial markets in the way that the models of the generation equity writers hypothesize.

In practice, the generation equity debate only has meaning within the very tightly drawn context of the pension and tax systems of individual countries. It is only within these very limited parameters that hypothetical balance of cash transfers can be calculated and efforts made to project them forward. When the concept is applied more broadly to society it immediately runs foul of the extreme complexity of assessing costs and benefits, and fairness, between different historical epochs. Even if in some sense cash thirty years ago can be equated with cash in thirty years' time, should not non-financial contributions to society enter the equation? How do you balance the contributions to society of those who fought in the Second World War and those who prospered in the peace? Do you calculate costs and benefits on the same index for those who fought on the losing side?

The key thrust of the debate is conservative (Walker 1990a). It rests on an individualistic view of society and responsibility that would prefer to see the state have no role in the transfer of resources. Pensions should be left to the private market. The *raison d'être* of the debate is clear when looked at from both sides of the Atlantic. The American social security system, because it is in a relatively early stage in its development, generates a fiscal surplus. This surplus has not been used to benefit future generations of elderly, it has been used to fund the federal budget deficit, especially the subsidizing of current government expenditure at the expense of future contributors to the social security fund. In Britain the opposite is true. The social security income from National Insurance does not cover the payments made under the scheme and the difference is made up from general taxation. Thus, although current taxpayers and future pension beneficiaries are in logically opposite positions in Britain compared with the USA, in both countries the generation equity argument is advanced. What is at issue is not fairness between generations but the redistributive role of the state.

The prudential life-course account suggests that we in the current generation making decisions about pensions in terms of contributions and benefits should make careful and cautious decisions about the future, rather than merely hoping for the best. These decisions clearly contain a large degree of uncertainty about the state of the future economy and current decisions should deal with this uncertainty by risk sharing: each generation taking an equitable portion of the risks involved in perpetuating a stable pension system, and the current generation not loading the risks forward to future generations. This should involve sensible reserves, sensible investments and not raiding assets for short-term consumption which would leave successor generations at greater risk of default on pension expectations. For the generational contract to be sustained, it is argued that there must be a measure of trust and solidarity across the generations, and that if the imperfections in the system are to be tolerated and seen as unfortunate rather than exploitative, justice must been seen to be done by each cohort. What the advocates of generational justice fail to see is that such solidarity is not achieved through some mythical compact between cohorts. Rather it is achieved through very concrete interpersonal relationships between old and young in families, communities and other basic social institutions. Although some authors are dismissive of intergenerational transfers within the family, there is clear evidence that, in general, families are flexible, adaptable and keen to meet their obligations (Finch 1987, Mayer & Wagner 1993: 523).

The nature of reciprocity between generations can be illuminated by the response from parents of children with a terminal illness. The fact they do commit themselves materially and emotionally to their children is a clear indicator of the power of the downward obligation, related to the asymmetrical reciprocity between generations. Life debts for the support from parents are repaid to children. It is children with little or no parental investment who are more likely, when they become parents, to neglect or pass the deficiency care to their children. It is not parents who can anticipate no return from their children in old age, because they will not live that long, who withhold commitment and investment in their children.

The position of the Bosnian pensioners, whose pension system has – as a pay-as-you-go system derived from the German model –

survived two world wars and the establishment of two new states, is highly illustrative. Because the vast majority of people in Bosnia are not earning very much in the current conflict, the payouts to pensioners are pitifully low and not enough to sustain life. However, if and when order and a working economy is re-established, the reciprocal right enshrined in the system will ensure that the elderly pensioners will be able to participate in the revived prosperity. On the other hand, a fully funded system, one that is based essentially on savings, would be wiped out by the levels of inflation and the destruction of physical assets experienced in the former Yugoslavia. It is perhaps not surprising that attitudes seem to differ between Europe, which has experienced wholesale destruction and economic collapse owing to war, and the United States, which has not experienced invasion, territorial redistribution and systematic destruction of economic infrastructure in war. In other words, it may be that in the long term, and taking into account the full range of insecurities, relying on the social power of reciprocity and a collective sense of social responsibility is a stronger option than individual investment plans in funded pension schemes based on the concepts of private property. There is something very American about the generational equity debate which stems from the radically different North American experience, where there is a very long political continuity and where it is over a century since war crossed its territory. There, experience of social security is very new and limited while the European experience is that pension systems have frequently outlasted states and constitutions particularly over the course of two world wars. Given this history, it is not surprising that in America a greater proportion of people see their old age more reliably secured through private property and leave unquestioned the political underpinning of those rights than is the case in Europe.

Idea of a moral economy applied to the position of elderly people

Thus the question of generational equity and the position of elderly people in society is not simply a demographic or economic one. It is essentially a political and a moral question. Some important insights have been gained in recent American literature on the cultural and moral issues of an ageing population (Cole 1992, Moody 1992).

The idea of the moral economy draws on the tradition of historical scholarship as exemplified by E. P. Thompson. Thompson (1971) describes how nineteenth-century food riots were seen by the participants as a morally just response to breaches in the concept of a "fair price" for food based on custom and need. The idea of just price has a long history, the clashes took place as the idea of just price was being crushed and lost to market forces. The idea of non-market prices is also found in the anthropology of pre-capitalist economies, for example in the work of Karl Polyani (Polyani et al. 1957). Martin Kohli (1991) also uses the concept of moral economy and sees not a decline of the moral economy but a shift from a "just price" to a "just return for labour". There is no doubt that the idea of "a fair day's pay for a fair day's work" is a powerful one in our society.

The idea of a moral economy can be translated into a key concept when associated with the idea of the life course. That is to say the moral economy principle applies to life courses as well as days of work. A fair return for a fair life. This becomes a possible and indeed dominant attitude when living a full life span becomes a relatively predictable occurrence. The moral life course (Kohli 1986, Cole 1992) has clear religious roots but in the modern West it is an entirely secular concept. It holds that if you live a "moral life" – that is one of hard work, diligence to the best of your ability, not idling or squandering your resources – then you deserve to live decently for the entire span of your life, including a decent old age and a proper burial. Thus, the converse: to die unattended or in poverty at the end of a "moral" life career is seen as morally outrageous.

This "moral life course" as part of the modern moral economy is not the same idea as the prudential life course. That concept is based on the concept of a contract or a bargain, that which reasonable persons would have done to secure their own financially secure retirement, and the subsequent use of this standard to measure the equity of intergenerational transfer. The "moral life course" is the socially constructed expectation of standards of living of people with unspoiled social identities when they have finished their working lives. Note for instance the argument made for the compensation to elderly people faced with increased costs for heating with the imposition of VAT on gas and electricity. A senior member of the cabinet – Michael Heseltine, among others – argued that elderly people living on pensions and savings could not work harder or save more to meet this extra cost and, therefore, they had a moral case to be shielded from the full cost of the new tax. The concept of moral economy is a useful one for examining the place of consensual basis of reciprocal obligations not only in the attitudes towards and the treatment of elders in peasant societies, as discussed in Chapter 3, but also with the market economies of Britain, the USA and other advanced industrialized nations.

We might also pose the question of what might constitute a moral economy in a postmodern world. The idea of "postmodernity" suggests that contemporary changes in culture, production and philosophy are mirrored in a moral economy located in radical individualism and hedonism. The idea of a just price for labour would no longer be a dominant value, rather freedom of lifestyle unconstrained by the disciplines of production and consumption would be the desired option. The moral economy in the postmodern world is an amoral "nice work if you can get it" one, which permits freedom of lifestyle, but sees no necessary relationship between effort and reward.

There is thus an important issue that lies in the relationship between reciprocity, power and the moral economy. This bears directly on the position of elderly people in our current Western society and on the future pension and welfare provision of coming cohorts of elderly people. However, the issue is a broader one applicable to the task of understanding inequality. The generation equity debate takes a specific restricted view of reciprocity. This view sees reciprocity as delayed exchange; what is given is returned. There is a more inclusive perspective that would include indirect reciprocity, what is given in one direction is returned by another. Hence, in terms of generations, what is received from the preceding generation is returned to the following one. However, there is another form of reciprocity, which Lévi-Strauss (1969) calls generalized reciprocity in connection with kinship and marriage. In these circumstances there is a generalized expectation of generosity and a right to receive but no specific counting of who gives or receives. Many hunting and gathering societies organize the distribution of food in this way. Antonucci and Jackson suggest that people distinguish between immediate and life-course reciprocity (Antonucci & Jackson 1989). The moral economy approach to generational equity which takes an informed life-course perspective should identify equity with generalized reciprocity. In terms of marriage, if each family group decided to opt for direct reciprocity and only to give as many marriage partners as it received, the whole marriage system would break down. Our systems of values require that we give our children freely in marriage without expectation of return. It is only by *not* counting that the system works "fairly". This is a better model for generational equity than support for the elderly in our society being based on a morality of direct reciprocity and a calculus of individualistic self-interest. Equality is then about reciprocity but not in a narrow sense, and it might be that equality is more achievable concretely by not requiring a close and exact individual tally of costs and benefits! The concepts of service or trusteeship, for example, are useful ones when considering current generations' responsibilities for handing on a sustainable natural environment to the rest of mankind including future generations. Similar concepts can also be applied to the welfare and financial support relationships between generations.

CHAPTER SEVEN

Social theories of ageing

In looking at the academic literature on old age and elderly people, I developed a dissatisfaction that forms the intellectual and professional motivation for writing this book. The treatment of elderly people and the ageing process in contemporary social theory is extremely limited and the treatment of age as a basis for inequality in British sociological literature is almost non-existent. How have those studying elderly people and old age sought to explain the latter's social significance? In particular how, and to what extent, can we draw on these ideas to understand the issues of inequality? And is the inequality experienced by older people the result of mechanisms that also generate more general social inequalities? The major branches of social thought on ageing and inequality can be classified into the following broad social theories: social biology; disengagement theory; the political economy of old age; structured dependency; and age stratification. Issues of social biology were dealt with in Chapter 5. This chapter will concentrate on theories that have a social character rather than biological or cultural explanations.

Functionalist approaches to ageing

Matilda Riley characterizing the study of social gerontology in the 1950s and early 1960s in America felt that the subject was in an early formative state but had established three major generalizations (Riley 1988: 25). These were:

1. that childhood experience leaves an indelible imprint; there are psychological development processes that continue to affect people even into the last stages of life;
2. that modernization lowers the status of the elderly, modernization – seen as world economic progress following a superpower model – was taken for granted;
3. that in anticipation of impending death there is a mutually satisfactory process of disengagement from social relations on the part of both older persons and society.

This list fitted well with the dominant sociological perspective of the time that followed functionalist ideas and those of Talcott Parsons in particular. This approach saw society as a complementary set of social roles operating reasonably harmoniously in ways that ensured its continuation. These three themes of disengagement, of modernization and of psychological development have been the core of the functionalist approach to the study of old age. I have already briefly touched on modernization approaches in Chapter 3, discussing in particular how unilineal models of social change are unhelpful. In this section I will examine other aspects of functionalist theory to see how they explain the condition of old age, and assess what can be learnt, either in a positive or a negative sense, which will add to our search for an understanding of the social inequalities of old age.

Disengagement theory

The role adaptation model of old age was one of the earliest sociological formulations of the social process of ageing and is known as disengagement theory (Cumming & Henry 1961). This is essentially a functionalist analysis and despite its manifest limitations it has shown surprising resilience in that it is still discussed seriously in contemporary academic social gerontological textbooks (Bond & Coleman 1990, Fennell et al. 1988, Hooyman & Kiyak 1988). This persistence stems partly from a failure to find satisfactory alternatives. Significantly, it also stems from the widespread empiricist and welfare orientation in the subject that frequently leads unselfconsciously to functionalist premises. As a consequence of seeing themselves as practical problem solvers, such writers are inevitably led to consider the issues that first motivated the disengagement theorists, which are how to identify successful ageing in terms of the individuals' adjustments to their roles in society.

Functionalism is the view that society is analogous to a living organism and that it is made up of a structure of interconnected parts in which each organ or institution plays a role in the maintenance of the whole. The functionalist view of society suggests that the degree of cohesion of society is based around a central set of values, norms and expectations and that the institutions that form the structure of society comprise of roles (normative expectations of behaviour) that fit together. A role is the rights and duties expected of a particular social position, and the explanation of the existence of a social role is that it benefits, or at least sustains, society in some way. Disengagement theory suggests that ageing involves the gradual withdrawal by elderly people from social networks and from role obligations, and a complementary tendency for other people to lower their expectations of older people. So the elderly person both disengages and is disengaged from society. The process is seen to operate on three levels: societal, individual and psychological. At the societal level, the elderly must be eased out of roles in which they no longer function effectively in order that younger role players can take them up and society as a whole can continue to work efficiently. On the individual level, disengagement enables the elderly person to conserve diminishing energies by only fulfilling the role demands of a restricted number of roles and role partners. The third or psychological level of disengagement refers to an emotional adjustment to the preparation for death. Cumming & Henry (1961) published data from their studies during the 1950s on older people in the American city of Kansas which suggested that old people who were able to accomplish a degree of disengagement had aged successfully.

Modifications of the original disengagement theory suggest that in addition to the loss of roles there is a positive view that there are new and substitute roles available to replace those lost through retirement or widowhood. This reflects the view found in many social psychological studies, that a high degree of social involvement is associated with indices of high morale and of personal satisfaction among elderly people (Neugarten 1982: 41, Rudinger & Thomae 1990). This is a more positive formulation and can be less readily interpreted as justification to throw elderly people on to the scrap heap of life because of the social necessity of generational role change. Other writers have suggested the easily observed pattern of both selective engagement and disengagement, especially a changing pattern of roles associated with social ageing. Some roles cannot be replaced easily, such as that of spouse; others may be more or less willingly relinquished, such as those of workers engaged in unpleasant physical manual work; while yet other roles may expand. Typically, kinship roles become more significant in later life (Harris 1990). Grandparenthood is a growing role. Furthermore the kinds of roles that are available to elderly people are not simply a feature of the capacities of elderly people themselves, but they are significantly restricted by those roles that are permitted to them by society. The particular conditions of elderly people, their family circumstances, the nature of their social networks and community positions, together with social structural constraints, create parameters within which elderly "actors" can secure rewarding personal and social roles in old age.

Most of the criticism of this disengagement position centres on the obvious ageist stereotyping that is involved in the theory. The theory accepts the characterization of elderly people as incompetent role players subject to inevitable decline, and fails to query how or why such a typification should come to characterize approximately one-third of the anticipated life span. However, the power of the theory appears to lie in its conceptualization of a universal process that is inevitable and functionally necessary for all individuals and social systems. All societies logically have to have social mechanisms to deal with the fact of death. The logic of functionalism suggests that for roles which play a positive and social stabilizing part in society there must be some mechanisms for transferring them between generations or society will prove unstable.

There is clearly a functional necessity for society to adjust to the fact of death; that people die and leave their roles – in other words social reproduction. However, such universalistic prescriptions as disengagement theory are not usually very useful in understanding the range of variations in lifestyles of elderly people. This is primarily because these prescriptions are ethnocentric (viewed from the point of view of our own culture) and chronocentric (looked at from the point of view of our own time), they take no account of history and the historical change in roles of elderly people. Some versions of this role theory of adjustment to old age use exchange theory as it has been developed by Blau and others (Blau 1964). They see social interaction as basically exchange, exchange of "prestations"; communications in which people seek to maximize the benefits from any inter-action in terms not only of material rewards but also social prestige, self-esteem and psychological rewards. Thus the low status of elderly people and changing patterns of roles are explained by the lack of exchange value possessed by elderly people. From this perspective, they have nothing with which to bargain for care and respect, except perhaps that expectation of reciprocity for past favours. This view directs attention particularly to exchanges and dependency relation-ships within the family. These kinds of formulation simply fail to deal with the complexity of social ageing and are founded on ageist assumptions about the social worth of elderly people. They treat all elderly people as the same and have difficulty in accounting for the variation among the elderly in Anglo-American society, let alone the rest of the world.

Psychological approaches

There is a link between the significance and the use to which the psychology of ageing is put and functionalist role analysis discussed above. So that although these psychological approaches have little directly to say about inequality and old age, they do serve to indicate ways in which characterizations of elderly people can serve as ideolo-gies or charters which inform the ways in which institutions and powerful groups construct their attitudes and behaviour towards old people. Because the functionalist approach sees roles as produced by society and external to individuals (individuals merely slotting into pre-existing social positions with established rights and duties), it is necessary for such theorists to revert to a psychological level to explain why different people perform the role differently. Hence both psychological and functionalist theories stress the significance of socialization processes. At least one benefit of linking developmental psychology to the study of ageing is to break down static views of personality and hence strengthen the idea that elderly people are capable of psychological growth. Ageing is a social, physical and psychological process of change but not merely one of statis and decline.

Erickson (1963, 1982) is a key psychologist noted for the idea of the developing stages of the personality through life. Table 7.1 is a version of his model of the eight stages of psycho-social development.

Table 7.1 Erickson's life-course stages.

Stages	Psycho-social crises	Significant social relations	Favourable outcome
1. first year of life	trust v. mistrust	mother or mother substitute	trust and optimism
2. second year	autonomy v. doubt	parents	sense of self-control and adequacy
3. third to fifth years	initiative v. guilt	basic family	purpose and direction; ability to initiate one's own activities
4. sixth year to puberty	industry v. inferiority	neighbourhood; school	competence in intellectual, social and physical skills
5. adolescence	identity v. confusion	peer groups and outgroups; models of leadership	an integrated image of oneself as a unique person
6. early adulthood	intimacy v. isolation	partners in friendship; sex, competition, co-operation	ability to form close and lasting relationships; to make career commitments
7. middle adulthood	generativity v. self-absorption	divided labour and shared household	concern for family, society and future generations
8. the ageing years	integrity v. despair	'mankind'; 'my kind'	a sense of fulfilment and satisfaction, (with one's life) willingness to face death

Source: Erickson 1963, modified in Hilgard 1979: 95, quoted in O'Donnell 1985.

This psychological view of the life course is particularly useful because it does not see personality as an object fixed in childhood never to change. However, it is possible to observe in this dia-grammatic representation of the idea of stages of psycho-social development a strong emphasis on young rather than the mature personality, which is characteristic of psychology as a discipline. Five of the eight life stages are pre-adult. Further no differentiation is made in later life, for example, between what are called the "third" and "fourth" ages by Laslett (1989). Therefore the schema has chronocentric features. Implicitly the life cycle is seen from the penultimate stage, middle adulthood, tacitly recognizing the power and status of people in this stage in setting societal values. It is also chronocentric because it does not take account of historical changes in the significance and problematic status of different life stages. Ado-lescent crises and "mid-life" crises, for example, have developed as features of modern Western society (Hepworth & Featherstone 1982, Hepworth 1987). The scheme is also ethnocentric in that it is based on the Western cultural preoccupation with the individual and can only be understood within the dominant cultural patterns of our cur-rent society. There is a further distortion in that the schema is also androcentric, for example career appears to be more important than motherhood in terms of "favourable outcomes" and there seems to be a male orientation in significant social relations. This structure of personality development might seem less plausible, and its "taken-for-granted" position more obvious, if the prime focus of discussion were non-Western women, for example Yanomami women (Donner 1982, cf. also Lizot 1985 and Chagnon 1977) or Hausa women (Smith 1954).

Life careers

The concept of life career has proved useful in trying to link the insight of continuing psychological development through life with the sociological patterning of the life course through sequential role changes. The idea is to look at the structure of roles, not simply in later life, but to see ageing as part of a whole life-time's career, in which preceding roles to some extent shape the possibilities for the next stage. The individual life is identified as a series of interrelated careers with transitions, successes and particular patterns of development. So throughout life, there may be a developing job progression, a change in family roles and a history of religious training and practice, which is continuous over a life-time. Thus later life is a culmination of some careers and the development of others and, either voluntarily or compulsorily, the end of yet other sequences: for example, children grow up and leave home, retirement terminates the major occupational career, imminence of death may provoke more rigorous ritual observance. This approach has been most developed in the psychological literature (Baltes & Baltes 1990) but the idea of a career is a useful sociological tool with which to conceptualize the sequencing of roles through a life course. It is useful because it contains three key ideas: first, the idea of voluntaristic action, people choosing various courses of action and new roles; secondly, the structural dimension by which society limits the choices available; and thirdly, the dynamic sequencing of elements whereby the consequences of previous actions get played out in the subsequent possibilities for choice and action.

These approaches to ageing from a functionalist perspective all take the roles and the expectations of elderly in society as something fixed and determined in the social structure. Those writers studying old age from a phenomenological or social interactionist perspective are much more concerned with what old age *means*. They ask: How is the meaning of "age" or "ageing" in particular situations socially constructed? This approach sees interaction as a process that generates meaning. In other words, the position of the elderly in society is created through sets of interactions such that some people in some situations are defined as "old". Thus a social situation may be totally age irrelevant, the ages of the participants may carry no meaning at all. However, age may become significant at the point at which the actors define the situation as age related and use the criteria of age to structure their understanding of what is happening. As, for example, when a 70-year-old in an old people's home says how she likes to pass the time by looking after the old people meaning the 80-year-olds.

Age stratification theorists

The United States has been a major source of sociological innovation in the period after the Second World War and has seen the greatest attention to theories of old age and inequality. In particular Matilda Riley has been a focus of an approach known as age stratification theory. Riley's approach is not classically functionalist but she shows clear signs of having developed her sociology in an America dominated by the sociology of Talcott Parsons. Riley's approach starts from the functionalist tradition but builds further by drawing on what would be seen from a European perspective as a Weberian approach to stratification. Riley accepts criticisms of functionalist theories which because of their emphasis on consensus and social equilibrium present an inadequate view of conflict and change. Riley's age stratification model assumes a system with inherent tendencies towards disintegration (in which sources of integration have to be explained). From the point of view of seeking to understand the relationship of age to inequality, Riley's work represents a number of significant steps forward. She systematically examines how the life-chances of people at different ages vary and demonstrates the division of society into age strata (Riley 1979, Riley et al. 1983, 1988a, 1988b).

One of the age stratification theorists' major contributions has been to systematize the use of the concept of the cohort into sociological theory and to link the idea of cohort succession to movements of historical social change. Riley points out that the members of a particular cohort develop biologically, psychologically and socially over time. They move together through the stages of family life, school grades, career trajectory, into retirement and ultimately death. They are constantly being reallocated to new sets of roles and resocialized to perform them. Thus movement between these age strata with increased years occurs partly by individual choice but it is also channelled by the age-related rules, linkages and mechanisms giving role sequences within the social structure and also conditioned by large social forces (like wars, depressions, cultural developments) that impinge on role sequence. In the flow of successive cohorts, each lives through a unique segment of historical time and confronts its own particular sequence of social and environmental events and changes. Society changes, and therefore people in different cohorts age in different ways. The ageing process itself is altered by social change (Riley 1988).

These two patterns, one of age strata, the other of cohort succession, are interlinked in complex ways. Cohort differences in ageing are socially dynamic because any major changes affecting one cohort have consequences for the next and subsequent cohorts.

Declines in mortality and changes in the standard of living, education, childbearing and health, affecting cohorts across this century have structured the circumstances of succeeding cohorts. A century ago over three-quarters of a cohort died before reaching adulthood; today over three-quarters of a cohort survives to at least age 65 and increasing proportions make it to age 85. The consequences of this increased longevity are various and complex. It allows education to be prolonged, and perhaps this is one reason why each successive cohort has experienced certificate inflation whereby the certification required to gain access rights to a job or profession are higher for each succeeding generation. Changes in family role relationships in one cohort produce implications for kinship in successive cohorts. Among couples marrying a century ago in America, one or both partners were likely to have died before the children had grown up; nowadays (if not divorced) they can anticipate surviving together for an average of 40–50 years. Today parents and children share a longer period of their lives as adult age-status equals than they do as adult and dependent child. In 1900 more than half of middle-aged couples had no surviving elderly parents, while today half have two or more parents still alive. Hence the grandparents in current cohorts born after the Second World War are able to have more influence on the lives of their grandchildren than those born a hundred years before.

Members of successive cohorts age in new ways, and so contribute to changes in social structure. This interplay between ageing and social structure can be illustrated through changing patterns of work and retirement. People's work experience has changed as the employment structure has changed. Increasing numbers of professional workers mean that career patterns change and include for example prolonged periods of training. This in turn eventually leads to better-educated elderly people who thus experience old age differently to previous cohorts. A cohort's response to social change itself exerts a collective force for further change. To continue the professionalization argument, better-educated and professionally trained elderly people may well lead to more articulate and powerful pensioner pressure groups who are effective in reducing the exclusion of elderly people from many areas of social life including that of employment. In family life there have been increases in divorce and remarriage that, combined with increasing longevity in modern cohorts, convert the current kinship structure into a complex matrix of latent relationships among dispersed kin and step-kin among whom ties of

160

solidarity must be achieved rather than taken for granted (Riley et al. 1983, Finch 1989). As one cohort presses for adjustments in social roles and social values, they influence other people throughout the age strata and contribute to continuing interaction in both ageing and social structure (Riley 1988: 30).

The human life span sets a rhythm of succession into sequential age roles across the life course and the inevitable succession of generations, but social change has no such in-built rhythm. Social change can be slow, fast, revolutionary or even unnoticed or denied. Society, therefore, is not only composed of successive cohorts of individuals who are themselves ageing in new ways, but these cohorts are continually forcing other cohorts to adjust their roles in the social structure. This flow of cohorts connects the two dynamisms of ageing and social change. The life-chances of one cohort structure the life-chances of others. The asynchrony between the pace of historical change and the rhythm of succeeding generations creates a further dynamic for change. For example the current younger generation in Africa saw their parental generation experience rapid and long-range social mobility following decolonialization, which created expectations for their own advancement. However, the recent history of population growth and economic stagnation has frustrated many of these expectations held by younger Africans. This frustration will itself be a force for change in Africa in the future. It is possible to see these complex relationships between cohorts as an example of the more general long-range social process of interconnectedness that forms the core of the work of Norbert Elias, which is discussed at length in the next chapter.

This age stratification approach does not use stratification in a "hard" sense, that it is used more generally in this book. The use of the term is more akin to the Weberian concept of "status groups" than as specific groups with objective common interests. Thus, although we must take from Riley the analysis of cohort dynamics and its ability to link personal experience of life course with historical change, we need to find theories that offer a more substantial explanation of how social inequalities associated with age are generated and how ideologies (the ideas and justifications of these inequalities) arise. A theory is needed that goes beyond a description of *how* age stratification works its way through society to *why* such processes occur, and includes a theory of history that explicates the direction of the social trends in society.

The political economy of old age

The political economy of old age in Britain is particularly associated with the work of Alan Walker and that of Chris Phillipson (Phillipson 1982, Phillipson & Walker 1986). There has been a considerable development of such approaches under the heading of "critical gerontology" both in Britain and the USA (Cole 1993, Minkler & Estes 1991). This has been the most fruitful method of considering the relationship between old age and inequality but it has a number of distinct problems.

Political economy can be understood to be the study of the interrelationships between polity, economy and society or, more specifically in modern society, the reciprocal influences between government, economic institutions and interests, and social classes and status groups. The central problem addressed by writers using political economy perspectives is the manner in which the economy and polity interact in a relationship of reciprocal causation affecting the distribution of social goods. Or, expressed in another way, the analysis of systems of production and distribution of social surpluses, and the justifications for that distribution. Marxism has been the dominant political economy approach, and despite its limitations the whole body of thought should not be simply abandoned merely because of the political and economic failure of Russian and East European regimes who also used that label for themselves. As long as we use the Marxist intellectual tradition as one among a number of possible methods, rather than as a self-justifying procedure to avoid an open critical use of the intellect, we can retain its powerful insights into the nature of inequality. Marxist analyses of old age are limited not because the methodology is weak but because they have never really been done effectively. The political economy of old age can provide the useful function of revealing the limitations and class biases of previous formulations of the place of elderly people in society and reveal the ideological nature of current perceptions of elderly people. However, it has proved more difficult to conceptualize a positive role for elderly people within this framework. Both the economism of early Marxist theory and practice and the emphasis on social reproduction that is more characteristic of present-day socialist feminism have had the effect of marginalizing elderly people. Emphasis on the revolutionary potential of, on the one hand, producers (male industrial proletarians) and, on the other hand, reproducers (women engaged in the task of family socialization) has inevitably reinforced the image of elderly people as redundant as agents of radical change and without a historically significant role. It is possible to suggest additionally that the Marxist tendency to equate the issue of ethnicity with that of migrant labour has a similar effect marginalizing the social significance of ethnicity and race in creating radical social change. How can the role of elderly people be reconceptualized from a radical perspective in a way that does not leave them on the sidelines of society? Is it really possible that 20 per cent of contemporary society can be lightly dismissed as historically irrelevant?

Low social status for elderly people is not the inevitable outcome of a natural process of ageing but is socially structured, and hence potentially open to change. In this process of inequality the state plays a large part in determining the events in the latter half of life which promote dependence, poverty and isolation among elderly people. What is meant by "the state" is not just the elected government of the day but that ruling complex of central administrative, legal, economic and political institutions that have become established over a long period of time, and that govern the scope and in large measure the nature of everyday social activities. A concept such as "structured dependency", which Phillipson and Walker sought to elaborate, is required to understand such developments in modern society. Otherwise some state policies are liable to misinterpretation as contributing to an enhancement of the welfare of elderly people when the real direction of change is more complex.

The logic of capitalism, which requires labour practices to be subordinate to the imperatives of a maximal return on capital, turns retirement into a reserve army of labour, a set of cheap easily manipulated workers who can be incorporated into the labour force at times of labour shortages but removed from the workforce at times of slump. Thus changes in retirement policies can be used under capitalism to change patterns of labour, expelling unwanted skills, undermining traditional work practices and increasing labour competition to keep the price of labour down. Thus there are two views of elderly people as an ex-proletariat. They may be either an alienated group, functionless and marginalized because they play no part in social production; or, alternatively, they might be an exploited group denied the product of their life-time's labour, poor not because they are at the sides of society but because they have been, and still are, fully incorporated into exploitative relations. Paralleling these alternatives are two versions of the welfare state, one as a bargain struck through the achievements of organized labour which provides a share of society's production for elderly people, the second as part of a manipulative strategy by which capital secures a minimum of political loyalty and minimizes potential social disturbance (see Ch. 6).

The elderly thus experience the dominant ideology of capitalism through the interpretation of work as opposed to idleness as meaning paid as opposed to unpaid labour. Retirement has then many of the attributes of unemployment. The loss of work by retirees is frequently experienced negatively, not only as an anomic response to the social isolation from the integrating role of work but also as a loss of sense of worth and contribution to society. This is particularly true for men in the past, because of the more restricted range of socially acceptable domestic roles available to them. There is an acceleration in mortality shortly after retirement, and indeed pre-retirement counselling has been found to have some effect in preparing workers for the adaptation needed on retirement and thus lessening the rates of suicide and mental illness. However, the root cause of such problems is not with age or retirement but with the ideological denigration of non-wage workers as unproductive parasitical kinds of people.

The ideological nature of the view of retirement as loss in Western society can be seen by comparing the ideologies of capitalism and those of lineage society (see Table 7.2). Lineage societies are found in horticultural or pastoral modes of production in which kinship provides the rationale for the membership of lineages that constitute property-owning corporate groups.

Ideologies from the right that stigmatize the non-employed, including the elderly, as unproductive usually use epithets like "feckless" or "scrounger", which imply moral blame to explain poverty or deprivation. However, the middle class in Western society is at little risk of poverty, as high earnings, fringe benefits, job security, the incremental rise of the typical salary profile and the consequent relative ease of individual "planning" and saving; all confer relative security and thus enable self-images of prudence and moral and financial rectitude to be maintained. Property ownership gives an added dividend and a degree of insulation against inflation. Although the "genteel poverty" (found in places like the backstreets of Hove or Worthing where savings were insufficient for a long-lived widow, and the capital in the property cannot be realized) illustrates that

Table 7.2 Types of ideology.

Individualist	Collective
Capitalist ideologies	Kinship ideologies
Individuals responsible for their own destiny, hence they are blameworthy when they fail to provide for themselves and show a lack of foresight in preparing for old age. Hence poverty brings dependency and low status with age	Kin are mutually responsible for the wellbeing of group members. Elders are valued for their collective contribution to juniors and hence are respected and have high status
Labour is a commodity, poverty and propertylessness function to ensure labour discipline and keep workers working	Labour is attached to land by family ties, and kinship obligations function to keep workers working

property ownership has its own problems. Structural dependency of elderly people results from restricted access to a wide range of social resources particularly income.

The competitive priorities of capitalism as a productive and social system means that it is unlikely to meet the needs of elderly people on a long-term basis. This incompatibility is manifest in four ways (Phillipson 1982: 3–4):

1. With each recurring recession it is the weakest sections of those who make up the workforce who are forced into redundancy and early retirement. This has the effect of shifting the balance of power and rewards from labour to capital, and the retirees lose out in pensions and public resources.
2. The priority given to maximizing returns on capital produces a distortion in the socially identified needs of elderly people. An example of this process lies in the medicalization of elderly people's problems and presenting them as having technical solutions, such as more drugs from which profits can be made. The dominance of capital means that the identification of people-centred problems with social solutions is less likely to be at the top of the social agenda.
3. The commodification of labour has the effect of breaking up communities and families through migration, the consequences of which for elderly people have been discussed in earlier chapters. The commodification of people and their relationships is to

the detriment of the social obligations to the elderly and the ability of family and neighbours to supply them.

4. Exploitation leads to poverty and thus deprives elderly people of the choice of desirable or fulfilling ways of living. Some of these mechanisms of exploitation that are particularly relevant to elderly people are discussed in Chapter 5.

There is also in America active advocacy of a political economy of old age (Cole 1993). Carroll Estes and Meredith Minkler are among the leading American analysts in this field (Minkler & Estes 1991). These writers suggest that the perception of the problem of poverty in old age is constructed by the administrative action of the state. Although there are considerable problems with satisfactorily measuring poverty, it is clear that the elderly in America are still disproportionately poor compared to the rest of the population. The poverty criteria adopted by government are constructed for particular purposes such as the supply of public benefits – for example Medicaid – and thus the definitions of poverty are enacted to ration access to social security payments. Minkler (1991) suggests that there are very many elderly people, in proportions larger than other sections of the population, with incomes just above state poverty lines. There are poor young people as well, but the idea of large numbers of elderly people depriving children of benefits is false. When discussing "the new victim blaming", Minkler sees the social problem of generational equity as arising not because of the existence of such inequity or from a sense of injustice but rather because administrations have budget problems. The administrations then seek to redefine their fiscal problems in a way that excuses their handling of economic issues and falsely identifies the victim of changes in government finances as the cause. Locating the issue of poverty and generational justice in the conflicts over federal budget expenditures (Minkler 1984) reveals how key interests place the priority for arms over support for the elderly, support for guns and military expenditure before hospitals and Income Support for both children and old people.

Structured dependency

A major attempt to develop a political economy of old age was conducted by the critical gerontologists in the early 1980s, of which

Phillipson's (1982) work was a particularly well-developed account. The essence of this critique was the idea of dependence. This was not the idea of dependence as developed by dependency theory although it could well have been influenced by it. Dependence is seen as the product of the bourgeoisie and the bourgeois state in that it curtails the autonomy of elderly people, requiring them to depend on the state through pensions and welfare payments and on welfare professionals who control and determine the "needs of the elderly". The government action to expand privatized welfare, including residential care, created markets for the entrepreneurs in care, and state "welfare" created a set of dependent client groups who could be used in the political and economic interests of capital, groups of professionals and bourgeois political parties. Phillipson thus takes the view that, rather than concessions squeezed from a reluctant bourgeoisie, pensions, health services and other features of the welfare state are part of the bourgeois conspiracy that manipulates the state to create the best available conditions for capital accumulation (including the political stability and lack of a unified working class that this requires).

"Forms of institutionalised ageism have been developed to suit the management of industry and the economy in capitalist and state socialist societies alike, and has come to be reinforced by the shifting social distribution of power." (Phillipson & Walker 1986: 43)

Phillipson sees old age as socially constructed and therefore, in a class-based society old age is experienced by the working class in specific ways. The analogous point can be made that experience in a patriarchal society also differs between men and women, and thus age will be experienced differently by the genders. The ideological construction of old age in a class-based society is seen as directly reflected in a range of welfare policies and practices including the ways in which the elderly are responded to by doctors and social workers. The role of the state is significant in the ideological construction of old age and in the production of dependency in elderly people. The state has a role in creating greater and artificial dependency that in turn has the effect of producing negative status evaluations of elderly people. In contrast, where the state has limited control in the private sphere of the family, elderly people have relatively high esteem in their roles of fathers, mothers and grandparents. There are two views as to how the state has this effect. First there is the view that the state is essentially an agent of capitalism merely reflecting the interests of business and secondly that the state constitutes an independent source of power based on institutional organization and that is legitimized through various ideologies. Each perspective identifies those who have an interest in the dependency of elderly people with a rather different emphasis. Those who see the state having a relatively independent role will stress the way in which giving pensions enables the state to take a paternal role and increases its legitimacy and thus its power. Further the adoption of professional roles and power relations enables state officials to attract personal income and status from their relationship to elderly people. Those who see the state merely as an agent of capitalism will identify issues associated with control of labour and capital as more crucial.

> In advanced capitalist societies, the social production of marginality and dependency in the later phases of the life cycle may serve a function in terms of . . . removing excess manpower from the competition for jobs, and as a foundation for the generation of large investment pools providing capital funds for both the private sector and the state . . . . Moreover, by fostering dependency on the state, people are induced to grant legitimacy and stability to the state as guarantor of the future security. (Marshall 1981: 98–9, quoted in Phillipson 1982: 158)

The "industrial medical complex" has also been the focus of analysis for the American political economy school (Estes et al. 1993, 1984). This school argues that the interests of business and the interests of professional medical and social worker come together in the creation of a market of dependent elderly for their drugs, hospitals, residential homes and other services. The power of these interests disables elderly people by removing their autonomy, defining their needs for them and redirecting the very large sums of public and private finance in ways that increase profitability and job security and status.

There are, however, further questions that stem from these perspectives. Both capital and labour have interests in the labour market and in manipulating the supply of labour to adjust the price of wages. How are these struggles reflected in the way in which elderly people are treated and the way old age is constructed ideologically? Pension funds have an important role as a pool of investment funds within modern capitalism. It may be argued that there is a process of socialization of capital through pension funds, such that more and more capital becomes part of the property (although not directly under the control) of the mass or at least a large number of people. Conversely there is a strong case for suggesting that the growing significance of pension funds is simply an alternative method of accumulation for a capitalist class. Comparison can be made here with the idea of contradictory class locations suggested by Wright (1985) in that workers can have common interests with capital in so far as they are part owners of pension funds whose future yields depend on the return on capital. Most people in Britain and Europe are, however, dependent on state pensions which, although they require contributions, are not fully funded schemes based on actual investments.

Perhaps the most important contribution of the structural dependency approach is the unmasking of the ideologies whereby the real physiological and biological changes that take place with ageing are utilized as a justification for denying old people the right to participate in discussions that affect them and generally to control their own lives (Walker 1987). The material and physical dependency of many elderly people is interpreted as "childlike" and used to justify treating them as if they were children. Furthermore, infantilizing the elderly eventually produces its own predicted result – old people may be induced to accept a childlike role as the only legitimate way in our society of being physically dependent on another person (Hockey & James 1993).

It is the argument of the critical gerontologists that the process of retirement, establishment of minimum pensions, residential care and the delivery of community services have created forms of social dependency among the elderly which are artificial. Forms of institutionalized ageism have been developed to suit the management of industry, professional bureaucracies and the economy and these have been reinforced by the shifting social distribution of power. This conceptualization is very hard for some people to accept. On the one hand, there has been abundant evidence of strongly motivated concern about retired, and particularly infirm, people; with many speeches being made about a caring, compassionate society and a flow of special measures and subsidies for the elderly section of the population. On the other hand, retirement incomes have been kept far below average earnings and there is continued pressure to reduce the average retirement age further and conversely raise the age of pension entitlement. There are continuing tendencies to segregate the frail and even the physically active elderly; and within community, as well as in residential, services there are tendencies to reinforce the dependent and non-participative status of the elderly. The rhetoric of choice which accompanied the first attempts to use public benefits to buy private care in Britain has been replaced by finance-driven assessments by social work professionals. "An artificial dependency is being manufactured for a growing proportion of the population at the same time as measures are being taken to alleviate some of the worst effects of the dependency. This paradox deserves to be understood and argued about more passionately than it is." (Phillipson & Walker 1986: 43)

What Phillipson and the critical gerontologists were trying to do was the very laudable aim of recapturing from the right the rhetoric of individual choice. However, as the 1980s moved on and the free market ideologies have taken their toll, it does not seem very plausible to look at the welfare state as a capitalist conspiracy to control labour when such determined efforts are being made to undermine it. The attack on the value of the state pension in Britain does not appear to fit the model of a strategy of creating dependency in the elderly.

Americans writing on the political economy of old age have raised issues about race and age. Minkler (1991) examines that which some researchers in California have called the coming race/age war; apocalyptic demographic ideas based on the varying ageing and fertility rates of different racial groups in California. There, as in Florida, elderly people are predominantly white, while the young workers include a much higher proportion of people of Hispanic or other minority origin. Conflict is predicted as a result. However, the reality of opinion expressed through surveys is that the young people and minorities in particular support social security measures. This is perhaps unsurprising as they depend on it more. Further, these minorities have the highest rate of ageing (because of rapid declines in fertility rate). Minkler & Estes (1991) have sought to challenge the myth of the homogeneous elderly and believe that political economy has helped to explain variation in the treatment of the old and has explicated the influence of race, class, gender and labour market condition on ageing.

Conclusion

It has been suggested that there has been a dialectical progression advancing the understanding of the social position of the elderly. The original thesis was provided by the first generation of social gerontological theories such as disengagement and activity theories. These approaches, as outlined above, are individualistic and psychological in orientation. The antithesis came with second-generation theories such as age stratification and structured dependency, which saw elderly people within a social structural framework and within a modernizing context. The third-generation or synthesis theories are theories that can bridge both structure and action (Hendricks & Leedham 1991). This synthesis is the kind of theory which this book seeks to define.

From the political economy approach we can take the ideas of the dynamics of age stratification and of structured dependency as useful ideas in understanding the relationship of old age and inequality. However, there are a number of significant problems with the theoretical position of the political economy of old age. The first is that it tends to subsume old age disadvantage under the mechanisms of class; and while it is clearly true that class fundamentally affects the condition of elderly people, it is also true that all inequalities cannot be reduced to that of class. Old age, race, gender and probably other unequal conditions need to be united with a theory of class, not subsumed as a mere branch of it.

The second limitation stems from the need to take account of the whole of people's lives when considering inequality, in other words to take a life-course perspective. People at different points in their life course have different relationships to capital, they may be employed and directly exploited through wage labour, or it may be exclusion from the labour market that is the source of their inequality. The life-course differences between generations need further analysis in political economy terms. The experience of class, as a real historical force located in the life of the workplace and communities, and the accompanying sentiments of class loyalty and solidarity are specific to different cohorts. E. P. Thompson (1968) points to the traditional or pre-industrialization sources of solidarity and resistance in the "making of the English working class". Just as the cohorts who experienced capitalist industrialization in Britain used values and symbols from their past to deal with the new situation, some currently living cohorts draw on their differing past experiences to make sense of and resist threats to their interests and welfare. For example, the organized pensioners' movement in Britain draws heavily on former trade unionists.

It is necessary to add a cultural and moral dimension to the political economy approach. It needs a critical moral dimension based on an appreciation of historical and cultural variability. Some versions of the political economy approach have tended to be mechanistic and treat culture merely as a reflection or by-product of social structure. They ignore the human elements of the historical process, the unpredictable and highly contingent elements of human action. Political economy theory needs rooting in a humanistic morality. Cultural questions about individuality, subjectivity, spontaneity or morality are not simply "dependent variables" to be explained by material factors (Minkler & Cole 1991). Concerns with justice, fairness, rights and obligations, which many Marxists rejected as aspects of liberal ideology, can serve positive functions (for example as a protection against certain forms of oppression) (Hendricks & Leedham 1991).

The limits of previous Marxist analyses of old age are to some extent challenged by those who developed the ideas of "structured dependency" and of a "moral economy". But the key question remains: How is it possible to conceptualize the position of old people without discarding the important insights derived from Marx on exploitation and class? I have suggested a series of ideas for a proper formulation of the relationship of age to the stratification system, and how elderly people fit into the patterns of exploitation in advanced capitalist societies. Still lacking, however, is a coherent conceptual paradigm for empowerment of the elderly. One way to explore ways to move from dependency to empowerment lies in Gramsci's concept of hegemony (Gramsci 1971). We need to understand how the dominant ideas in society can be radically reformed, how the social position of elderly people can be positively reconceptualized based on the moral and philosophical consent of the members of society grounded in their taken-for-granted cultural assumptions.

CHAPTER EIGHT

The reproduction of inequality: power, structured dependence and the life course

The purpose of this book is the sociological analysis of old age. In particular it seeks to understand how old age and inequality fit together in society. In order to do this it has been necessary to look not only at old age but at other forms of inequality and social differentiation as well. Sociology used to concentrate on the examination of class as the basis of inequality. But there is a growing consensus in sociology that replaces class as the central social process in advanced capitalist societies with a triumvirate of class, race and gender. Some of this writing that has sought to bring coherence to an understanding of inequality has been highly insightful. For example, in the field of social policy, Williams has developed a view that the organization of welfare around work, family and nation reflects the structures of class, race and gender, which unfold in the context of the process of capitalism, patriarchy and imperialism (Williams 1990). What is particularly useful about this theoretical scheme is that it emphasizes that inequality is not a collection of attributes but a social process. In this attempt to regain a single theory of inequality, however, other systematic inequalities have been neglected. In particular that of age has not been sufficiently considered and this is a major inadequacy of many such tripartite formulations. What is now required is a unified approach; a single theory that accounts for not only these three very significant forms of inequality but in addition, all other possible inequalities as well. It is for this reason that the examination of old age is so essential, not only for the intrinsic interest in understanding a growing part of the life course but because any such unified theory of inequality must be able to account for age-based inequalities.

Limitations of gerontological theory or of sociological theory?

The lack of adequate theory in the field of social gerontology has been adversely commented upon on many occasions (Johnson 1978, Phillipson 1982, Fennel et al. 1988) and stems in part from the social policy orientation of much of the interest in the field. However, in thinking through the material for this book, I have become aware that it is as much the inadequacy of existing sociological theory in providing coherent accounts of old age in our society as a lack of interest in theoretical topics by social gerontologists that are responsible for this neglect of theory. Feminists trying to write feminist sociology, or at least produce a non-gendered sociology, and those trying to understand race and ethnicity have had to struggle with the limitations of existing sociological theory. It is not surprising therefore that when similar questions about power, stratification, structure and the social process of age-based inequality are examined, further limitations in social theory are revealed. However, and perhaps of greater importance, when such enquiries are made new insights become possible. Therefore the central focus of this book has been to draw on theoretical discussions in branches of sociology that have not previously been brought together and link the study of inequality, stratification, class, gender, race and ethnicity with the study of elderly people and the life course. This attempt has required a critical examination of the existing approaches to social inequality within sociology, as well as a review of the literature on old age and the life course. Further, it is clear that the study of old age can feed back and provide insights for our understanding of other inequalities.

It is not possible simply to combine the differing approaches to inequality in the different topic areas. Those writing on different aspects of inequality – class, race, gender, etc. – tend to acknowledge the existence of other forms of inequality but these tend to be treated as a residual category of "ideas that are also relevant". Adding "ageism" to a list that includes "racism" and "sexism" and other potential "-isms" is a very limited explanation of inequality because it locates the problem in individual attitudes. Such explanations are both too general and too specific. They do not explain the particular problems of specific groups of elderly people in villages, towns and cities across the contemporary world. Neither do they give an insight into the systematic variations in inequality between different societies or the patterns of social change that shape current possibilities.

Paula Dressel (1991), in "Gender, race and class beyond the feminization of poverty in later life" argues for a political economy of ageing but one in which race is the major determinant of poverty among American elders. She points out that the construction of the problem of elder poverty through the concept of feminization of elderly age groups has been widely accepted because such a position can create a wide coalition of political interests with which to tackle the problem. However, she argues that this approach might be a fatal remedy because it does not focus on the major cause of poverty that she identifies as race. In a powerful metaphor she states that the feminization of poverty has tended to be based on the "add and stir" approach to theory.

> Racial-ethnic women have not been overlooked in most writing on the feminization of poverty in later life. The tendency has been, however, to take the "add and stir" approach that leads to race-blind theoretical formulations. That is, what are meant to be general statements about gender and poverty are made and then, as after thought or elaboration, specialized statements about black (or Hispanic or native American) women are made. (Dressel 1991: 247)

The English cultural equivalent to the "add and stir" approach characterized by Dressel (1991) might be taken from Woolworth's sweet counter; the analogy of a "pick and mix" approach to theory seems to characterize attempts to link the different forms of social inequality. A bit of this, a bit of that, put together in the same bag, an eclectic collection of ideas without coherence. Or, to extend the culinary metaphor, theories are too frequently treated as a menu of categories; choose your own pizza toppings, take an idea from this tub with a slice of that concept in the hope that it all comes out crisp and wholesome. These analyses do not dispute that age, class, gender, etc. *should* be considered but rather that the problem is that they do not know *how* they should be considered. The key that is necessary to link the various forms of inequality is a theory of process. It is a coherent idea of how to do the cooking, not a list of possible ingredients that is required to go beyond the "add and stir" approach.

175

Social reproduction: differentiation and domination processes

The process that enables society to continue as observable patterns of behaviour is known as social reproduction. There are two kinds of process that enable society's institutions and ideas to continue despite the continual replacement of personnel; these are differentiation and domination. The distinction between patterns of social reproduction that lead to differentiation and those that lead to domination is of course essentially analytical. These concepts are tools with which to understand society. The relationship between them is intertwined in actual historical behaviour. Differentiation is a universal process and logically must occur prior to domination. However, because there is no starting or end point to society the social processes of differentiation and domination are in most societies so closely intertwined as to be difficult to separate. Differentiation is a universal process because society is not possible without it. Domination is nearly universal, but some societies are more successful at combating it than others. There are some small-scale societies in which many aspects of social life do not involve domination and there are some small parts of existing larger societies in which domination is not of great significance (Lee 1979, Turnball 1983, 1984). However, the great majority of social life can be considered as patterned by both differentiation and domination. Domination can lead to differentiation, and this process can be illustrated in the formation of some ethnic groups. Further differentiation can lead to domination; the whole discussion of the development of class structures can be used to illustrate this relationship. This analytical distinction is useful in so far as it enables us to think about issues of inequality in our societies which can encompass both the many distinctions, including gender, age, class and race – which structure our society – and also the different processes by which inequality is created, including those of imperialism, of nationalism, of capital and of family and kinship.

Social reproduction is both institutional and cognitive. I am not suggesting that this distinction between differentiation and domination coincides with the distinction between "cognitive" and "institutional". It is not that processes of differentiation are simply cognitive; thought processes by which categories of people are included or excluded. Nor is domination simply an institutional process made up of patterns of roles and social structures. Differentiation and

176

domination are in a different analytical dimension to that of the usual sociological categorization of roles into economic, political, cultural, social and religious institutions. These types of role may exhibit the consequences of the processes of differentiation and domination. Thus it is possible to conceive of processes of economic, political, or cultural differentiation. Cultural differentiation might be illustrated by how ethnic groups come to be conceptualized as different in terms of linguistic, religious or cultural symbols. Chapter 4 provides an illustration of how this is done for the category "old". Economic differentiation would be identified in terms of the division of labour and economic specialization processes, while political differentiation might be seen in terms of political roles and changing degrees of political specialization. On the other hand, domination as a different kind of process would suggest that cultural domination could include issues of hegemony; economic domination issues of exploitation; and political domination issues concerning force, military oppression and legal authority.

Processes of domination: exploitation and hegemony

It is possible if we take each pattern of inequality (class, race, gender and age) to see that for each there is a characteristic pattern of domination and of differentiation. However, we can also see that there are common elements in these two patterns. If we take class, the pattern of domination is usually called capitalism, and processes by which this form of domination has been reproduced have been discussed extensively and include processes of exploitation and processes of hegemony (the dominance of particular ways of thinking). If we look at gender, the pattern of domination is usually called patriarchy, but processes of exploitation and hegemony have also been used to explain this pattern of domination. The domination involved in ethnicity has been called nationalism or perhaps imperialism or racialism. Again in this case the reproduction of these patterns of dominance has been through exploitation, hegemonic domination and processes conceptually similar to those that operate for gender and class. If we then look at domination on the basis of age we can see that this can either be a form of patriarchy (as discussed in Ch. 5) and associated with the kinship order in society, or, in modern industrial society, it is more likely to be expressed as ageism. In Chapter 5 I illustrated how exploitation can be seen to work in the case of old age; and in Chapter 4, how the cultural/ideological construction of old age works and can thus also be interpreted as a hegemonic process. Both lead to domination.

We should perhaps note in passing that some have sought to make biologically based arguments for all these patterns of domination. Theories of natural difference leading to domination have been used in each case – to attribute the inequality to "natural" rather than "social" causes. Thus old people are naturally dependent because of their lack of power, poor health and disability. In terms of gender, women are naturally submissive while men are bigger, more powerful, more aggressive as part of their biological make-up. Racialist arguments are also constructed in a similar manner: lower IQ measurements; being better at sport; inability to invent square houses are attributed to the "natural" products of race. Even class, in terms of a natural meritocracy, can be justified on the basis of inherited intelligence and entrepreneurial attitudes. Although as an anthropologist I accept the need to incorporate biological and evolutionary arguments into the proper understanding of society, I hope I have indicated in the preceding chapters why these explanations are untenable.

Processes of differentiation: socialization and hegemony

The cues by which people are differentiated on the basis of age, gender, race or class are obviously not the same. However, the processes by which those cues are reproduced are very similar. So class differences, even though they are not "natural categories" but based on ownership of property or status distinctions made in terms of cultural capital, can be understood as generated in a similar manner to gender, race or age differences. These class distinctions are constructed and reconstructed by economic processes such as the division of labour and through patterns of socialization. If we look at gender, feminist writers have shown how gender is reproduced through socialization, and in addition through the economic processes of the division of labour – the same processes that reproduce status and property distinctions. Furthermore, with ethnic distinctions, studies have shown the importance of socialization in the immediate reproduction of prejudiced attitudes, yet also in this case the significance of the ethnic division of labour in creating and sharpening social differences is apparent. All the processes that have been seen to apply to class, race and gender are relevant to the reproduction of age-based distinctions. The different processes of differentiation – the division of labour, socialization of various kinds and ideological control of the dissemination of ideas – apply to old age. People learn to make distinctions between young and old in certain times and places by attending to certain cues and giving them particular social significance. The distinction "them and us", in terms of black and white or Catholic or Protestant, can be learnt and unlearnt, and people can come to "know" what the difference between male and female means. Indeed these differentiation processes interrelate because we have to learn that it means different things to be male and female at different ages, in different ethnic groups and classes. We learn "class" through the idea of property, differentiating what is "ours", and we learn status distinctions by coming to know what is whose.

We must not limit the processes by which people learn to "tell" socially significant differences to child socialization. Adult socialization of various forms plays a part in the boundary creation and maintenance processes differentiating social categories. For example, many studies of race and ethnicity show a continuing process of social learning, particularly as social distinctions and values change and elaborate through time (Banton 1987, Ringer & Lawless 1989). All these short-term, generation by generation, patterns of the reproduction of difference are complemented by the historical development of hegemonic ideas in longer cycles of social change.

Therefore the issues that we have been considering in this book – in other words, class, race, gender and age – are all the result of particular kinds of differentiation processes and particular kinds of processes of domination. The theme of how differences between people on the basis of ownership of property, gender, ethnic attributes and age are created and re-created is the centre of this book. Each of these cues to social difference are of course manifested in society through institutional arrangements. With class, there are institutions such as private property, the firm, the estate; with gender, institutionalization is in terms of family and household; with race and ethnicity, the state and empire are the key institutions; while for age, it is retirement and the institutions of the life cycle. Domination processes lead to the inequalities that we have noted which affect these categories, so that

Table 8.1 Patterns of inequality.

Differentiation	Historical process	Institution	Hegemonic relations	Exploitative relations
Gender	Patriarchy	Family	Sexism	Domestic labour, labour market segmentation and exclusion, consumer weakness
Ethnicity/race	Imperialism	Nation	Racism/nationalism	Imperialism; unequal exchange, labour market segmentation and exclusion, consumer weakness
Property	Capitalism	Class	Class ideology	Capitalism; wage labour, labour market segmentation, credentialism, unequal exchange
Age	Chronologization	Age strata	Ageism	Labour market exclusion, domestic labour, consumer weakness

types of domination – such as exploitation, coercion, legitimation processes and use of authority – are involved in all four of these types of inequality. These arguments are summarized in Table 8.1. However, this list (class, race, gender and age) is not definitive. There are many ways in which processes of differentiation and of domination can come together to create many other forms of social inequality in specific historical circumstances.

The processes of hegemony and exploitation listed in Table 8.1 should be seen as the principal or characteristic ones operating in the context of the particular institution but not as the only ones. The same relations can be seen to operate in all or most institutional forms, for example labour market exclusion or segmentation will have an effect on all the social categories listed. It is thus possible to perform the thought experiment of adding a further criterion X which differentiates people into unequal categories Y and Z by a process called X-ism and see if the kinds of processes and conflicts presented can accommodate this additional form of inequality. If we substitute a further likely candidate such as disability, the pattern seems to fit; if we try an unlikely hypothesis such as "cat lovers", the processes described appear to be irrelevant.

Generalized patterns of inequality

There are a series of standard questions that can be asked about any given social category. If we call that category x, we can ask what "x" contrasts with; we can further ask how x and non-x's are seen to be different and by what cues these differences are marked. Finally we can ask how that distinction is reproduced. The above discussion of socialization or economic differentiation processes illustrates some answers that may be found to this question. Then we can ask how patterns of domination reproduce the inequality between x and non-x's. Possible answers may be sought by looking at questions about exploitation and hegemony and other processes for the reproduction of domination. If we want to construct an argument about why being an x or not being an x is a significant feature of any society, we have to look at the longer-term trends in social reproduction in order to discover why particular patterns of differentiation and domination operated in a particular period.

However, what links the rows of Table 8.1 are life courses. The processes impinge on individual life courses in differential ways and at varying levels of determination. Historical social change is experienced by people through having their life courses structured in new ways. People also respond and react to these social pressures, they do not necessarily accept the inequalities being imposed upon them. All contemporary life courses have been structured in ways in which elderly people are more likely to be exploited and undervalued than cohorts who have not yet reached advanced years. It is the argument of this book that the idea of a structured life course provides the method of linking all various forms of social inequality. It can do this because the life course is something that is located in history, it changes in time with historical change. It is something that is bound and constrained by the material circumstances in which it is lived. There are many social changes that structure particular life courses: life-history processes, marginalization, job market processes, family processes, cohort processes, property rights, professionalization and disablement, among others. All life courses are conditioned by the large historical patterns of social change that are summarized in Table 8.1 as patriarchy, capitalism, imperialism, and chronologization. All these are processes which structure the life course. They have been discussed through this book and have been shown to have differential impacts on women as opposed to men, blacks as opposed to whites, elderly as opposed to the middle-aged.

There is a history to who is considered to be black, or a minority, or old and what those labels are taken to mean. It is clearly possible to examine these histories and reveal the nature of the categories that are used in society and describe how they have developed. It is a much greater problem to explain why those cultural patterns and changes occurred. They are not random events without causes. The starting point for such theorizing must lie in some material circumstance, and in the ecology of productive and reproductive relationships. The term "ecological" is used to indicate the intricate feedback loops that link together the stuff of history, the events, the ideas and activities of people. To develop an understanding of why inequalities have changed through history we need to look at issues of power.

Inequality and power

It is necessary to link together the two themes of social construction of identity and meaning and the production of inequality. This will produce both a better view of inequality and a better understanding of the social significance of age. Both these elements are required for an adequate theoretical formulation. Hence the stress in this chapter on social differentiation (which draws on the constructionist themes) and dominance (which draws on materialist themes). However, I do not see these two processes as independent and equivalent. The constructionist processes of differentiation take place within the historical sequence of life courses, they are therefore subject to power relationships – the patterns of domination that are historically received at any given time. The problem is specifying accurately the relationship between them.

Social inequality cannot merely be based on the social construction of meaning, we also have to appreciate the importance of power. To state that "Inequality is then about the social differences that are recognized in society and that are given a positive or negative value" – as I did in the Introduction – requires in addition a theory that specifies how differences come to be recognized and evaluated. The ideological impact is in the apparently impersonal "are given" phrase – buried in those words are the effects of power. Who in society has the power to have their definitions of categories accepted as positive or negative? In order to understand social inequality then, it is necessary to appreciate that power is embedded in social categories and social evaluation of categories, such construction of inequality does not happen in the abstract but is the result of the exercise of power by some people over others. The most useful kind of definition of power for the purposes of this book will require a materialist base, not merely cultural domination reflected in the ability to impose a definition of the situation. Such a purely constructionist definition would produce an unhelpful identity between differentiation and domination.

Power is a relationship. Power is not a thing – not like a sword or a bag of gold; it is a relationship between people. Power then is only ever a potential when future actions are to be considered, and only identified with greater certainty in the consequences of past action that can be examined and measured. All social relationships involve a balance of power. Domination is the unequal balance of power in a relationship. The chief characteristic of the relationship is a lack of reciprocity. This lack of reciprocity can be identified in material terms: who gets what out of the total social wealth generated through society. Power is the ability to have others act in one's own interests rather than their own. Dependence is related to powerlessness. Relationships of dependence constitute one extreme in a range of possible interdependences between people. Because power is never absolute, there is always – to some degree – mutual influence where power is concerned and thus there is always some balance of power in relationships however asymmetrical that balance may be. Such a relationship might be described as interdependence. However, where there is not only interrelatedness but also a very large differential in power, the label dependence is appropriate. Logically a third position can be conceptualized which is that of limited social interaction involving restricted mutual influence; a relationship of non-interdependence.

The concept of power should include not only the Weberian idea of the probability of obedience (Weber 1978) but also the ideological issues of constructing the agenda. Power is expressed through all processes by which collective interests become not simply identified and pursued but also may be systematically suppressed. Power lies not only in winning the public debate but also in keeping issues out of public consciousness and off the agenda. Is this why elderly people in Britain have not been noticeably vocal or active in asserting their interests politically (Midwinter & Tester 1987)? Steven Lukes (1974) suggests that a one-dimensional view of power focuses on political behaviour, decision making, observable and overt conflict. This one-dimensional view of power sees interests as policy preferences revealed by political participation. He also describes a two-dimensional view of power which identifies both issues and potential issues, overt and covert conflict, but still treats interests in a subjective way as grievances or preferred policies. Lukes' three-dimensional view of power is a thorough critique of the behaviourism implicit in the previous two approaches. It focuses on decision making and control over the political agenda, so that issues and potential issues and latent conflicts become legitimate areas of study. Interests are defined in an objective manner, recognizing that ideological blinkers may mean members of society are unable to articulate them. Power will be used in a manner that incorporates the way in which the control of ideas as well as control of physical force and other resources impact on people's material interests.

Interests in turn are a tricky concept. Interests may diverge between conflicting short- and long-term interests. There may be genuine ambiguity between ideas of what constitutes someone's best interests. People might not know what their interests are and it is possibly even more difficult for an outside observer to know what those interests are. Although we have to take account of the interpretation and negotiation of social meanings, behaviour, life chances and possibilities for action are structured by such things as class or age even if the actors involved are not conscious of there being classes or age groups, or of themselves as being a member of a class or an age group. For example, individuals living in a modern industrial society cannot escape the impact of levels of unemployment and the consequences this has for their own wage rates and employment prospects and opportunities. The market for labour exists independently of people's consciousness of being a member of the working class or any understanding of their labour market interests. By analogy, you do not have to think of yourself as old for the consequences of a social definition of old age to fundamentally structure your individual identity. For example, your life chances as an elderly person in the job market are structured, and even if you as an individual may have been fortunate in how those life chances have fallen out, your life is still structured by what has happened to others. The meaning of your identity as someone with a full-time job at 70 is inevitably coloured by the fact that so many others do not have such jobs. Common interests are real, even if we do not know what they are, because they are real in their consequences. Old people may have common interests intrinsic to a particular social structure, they may have such interests forced upon them by the actions of others, or they may create them for themselves. They may have objective common interests derived from their exclusion from the labour market even if they are not as individuals aware of this. They may have common interests imposed on them by the development of professions and the resulting dependency relations, or they may, by collective action, create a common interest in subsidized public travel or certain types of day-time broadcasting.

It is important that "the elderly" do not become a category outside of this discussion, incapable of expressing their real interests. Why are active organizations of old people not more in evidence? Where do they articulate their claim to equality and express a sense of inequality? There is a danger in this question of reinforcing stereotypes of the age, but it is nevertheless a highly significant question. There are clearly particular difficulties for the elderly to organize and express themselves. Many old people frequently deny that the negative stereotypes of old age apply to them, although they believe that they do apply to others. The conflicts are real but may well be hidden in the manner of Lukes' (1974) third notion of power, which suggests that there could be a kind of ideological blindness to the real interests of elderly people. There is an alternative possibility which is that the oppositions to inequality are expressed in ways that are not viewed as such.

Structured dependency and the life course

Structured dependency is a term used by the critical school of social gerontology, which contains the ideas of structure and dependency and can usefully be expanded and generalized. The creation of dependency – or perhaps "structuration" – does not just happen, it is done to some people by others. The idea of structured dependency, when linked to those of age stratification, life course and cohort succession, reflects a dynamic process, a process that explains how the reproduction of domination is achieved. With the notion of structured dependency we can fit together the various social processes that create social equality and think about them as facets of a single process. Unlike approaches that have taken the idea of social exclusion as the basis for stratification, structured dependency requires an active relationship. The relationships between groups are being structured, namely there is exercise of power in creating the terms of the relationship. That which is being structured is dependency, in other words a relationship of unequal power. Such relationships deny reciprocity and thus involve elements of exploitation. So structured dependency is the general process by which some groups of people in society receive an unequal share in the results of social production.

Thus we understand the social process of patriarchy, which largely but not exclusively takes place through familial and kinship institutions, as the creation of structured dependency of women on men. It is the structured relationship which undervalues women by attaching them to the undervalued domestic sphere and enables their labour, particularly domestic labour to be used non-reciprocally by others. Class relationships are those by which people with property and capital can structure the lives of others and non-reciprocally receive part of the value of their labour. Imperialism is the relationship that structures racial inequality and enables black people and other ethnic groups to be labelled as inferior and enslaved and exploited through institutions like plantations, migrant labour and sweat shops. The monopolization of professional knowledge and skills and their use to create dependency in elderly and disabled people in particular, and clients in general, is another facet of structured dependency. This too is a non-reciprocal relationship which structures an unequal distribution of social value. Even some consumer processes can be understood as structured dependency and as exploitative. With a sufficient degree of monopoly and power people can be made dependent on those selling or distributing certain products. The tobacco industry is a particularly clear example, highly monopolistic, it creates dependency to the point of addiction and is closely tied to the structure of the state. This is also the case with pensioners and the monopoly provision of utilities such as water, gas, electricity, telephones and housing which has been looked at in Chapters 1 and 5. It is not the possession of the characteristic female, old, black, working class, or whatever which creates the unequal relationships, it is utilization of these criteria by powerful people that creates structural dependency. For example, the effects of patriarchy are limited in adolescence in our society when familial ties are weak, although they are particularly oppressive in those societies in which adolescent roles are avoided to control female reproductive power through early marriage.

The terms life course and structured dependency can be usefully expanded considerably beyond their original use. Phillipson (1982, Phillipson & Walker 1986) took the material dependency that was the prime direction of Townsend's work and linked it to interpersonal dependence as a critique of professionalization. One meaning of structured dependency is, according to Phillipson, the sociological equivalence of learnt helplessness in psychology. By analogy, liberation from structured dependency involves self-help (although this self is likely to be a collective self). Thus Fennell (1986) is correct when he calls for not only theories of dependency but also independence. He suggests that elderly people are most likely to achieve independence when they have a variety of alternative resources on which to draw to meet their needs. A somewhat similar point is made by

Blaikie & Mcnicol (1986) when they examine the marginalization of elderly people. It is elderly people's marginal position in society, marginal to economic and employment structures, to family and kinship structures, which limits their range and choice of resources.

Much of this expanded concept of structured dependency is captured in the well-developed literature on dependency theory, which looks at relationships between the underdeveloped Third World and the dominant capitalist states of the West (discussed in Ch. 6). The centre–periphery model is not simply a geographical image, but stands for a social centre that has power and autonomy and a socially marginal periphery that has neither. There are both psychological and cultural aspects of dependency, and also material and exploitative aspects. The analysis of racism including work by Franz Fanon (1967, 1968) looks at the psychological as well as the physical domination created in colonialism. Much work, however, has gone into demonstrating the exploitative relationship between the Third World and the West and the methods by which the extraction of surplus value is achieved. The theory of unequal exchange suggests mechanisms by which the lack of choice and flexibility on the part of dependent economies (most crucially through colonial domination or neo-colonial clientship) can lead to exploitative exchange relationships – undervalued primary products or labour as opposed to overvalued manufactures, or technical and commercial expertise. Thus there is a direct parallel between the way in which the surplus value was extracted from colonial countries and used to build the industrial and commercial domination of the West, and the way in which those in retirement failed to reap the benefits of their productivity during their working lives and came to be dominated by the very institutions whose vitality they helped to generate.

Reciprocity as the basis of most social interaction and behind most moral precepts seems a good starting point for the critical analysis of society. If inequality is looked at as a failure of reciprocity, it is both a social and a moral concept (Turner 1986). Putting the two broadened concepts together, structured dependency applied to life courses, can lead to a critically enhanced understanding of inequality. The labour theory of value gives a method of understanding the distributive context of structured dependency – who gets what from whom. But the ideas of the life-course approach also enable a dynamic view of structured dependency because the balance of gains and losses does not remain constant. The effects of structural dependency change in systematic ways throughout the life course. The life course sets reciprocal exchange within a history and within a time frame; structured dependency sets such exchange within a framework of power. Different forms of inequality are reflected in different life courses. Both the cultural aspect of inequality, the historical changing sequences of ideas and meanings that divided and categorized people, and the material conditions of opportunity and exploitation can be contained within the one concept. To understand the unequal position of elderly people in the contemporary West requires therefore a full understanding of the sequences of life courses that make up that society of the kind discussed in Chapter 3. Thus for example the work on the history of the life course (Hareven 1982; Kohli 1986, 1990; Grillis 1987; Cribier 1989, etc.) in the last two hundred years in the West is a crucial commentary on the much more extended literature on the history of class over the same period. Such histories of class, of course, discuss issues of exploitation and hegemony. However, integration with a life-course perspective make the social and political movements more intelligible. It is possible to link the ideas of cohort succession to changing social and political conditions of exploitation, for example history of changes in capitalism, through the life courses of various groups and classes of successive generations. The concept of "life course" as opposed to "life cycle" has a historical component, the life course has date as well as age and chronological sequence.

The use of the concept "life course" should also be expanded. It started as a useful psychological tool revealing the way in which the personality continued to grow throughout life. One way it can be expanded is close to Weber's use of the term "life chances" to describe a key characteristic of stratification systems. The idea of the life course as a career, with varying chances or probabilities of material reward or lifestyle at different points, is a useful perspective. However, the idea of a life course can contain an important extra ingredient to that of the life-time career and that is "interconnectedness". Life courses need not be individualized but can be seen to contain webs of connectedness; individual life courses are located in networks, groups, institutions, generations and cohorts. The life course should not be dichotomized as either an individual or a collective phenomenon.

There is not a dichotomy between the "individual" and "society", they are each impossible without the other; they are abstracted aspects of the same thing (Elias 1978). It is sometimes difficult for those socialized in the highly individualistic cultures of the West to appreciate that the individual is just as much an abstract concept as society but nevertheless we should give no more analytical primacy to the idea of the individual than we should to social structure. The use of the concept of life course can avoid dehumanizing people as "individuals". An "old person" is only part of a person. People do not experience themselves as abstracted into age categories; a proper concept of an individual person should be the whole life course of that individual. Inequalities then lie between life courses. Thus people work, contribute to society and are exploited over the whole course of their lives not merely any particular part of it. Pension rights should belong not to the old as a category but to the person as a whole life course. They should be seen as a just and generalized exchange between people thought of as a whole life course, not as a special privilege granted to one section of society on the basis of age criteria. This formulation has the advantages of not segregating off the elderly as a separate category and identifying the whole issue of social transfers in terms of limiting exploitation across the life course and creating an enabling society that liberates people from socially structured constraints (which limits in particular the life-course possibilities of women, ethnic minorities, the disabled, etc.). This concept of a person as an individual life course also undermines the rhetoric from the right which talks of individual choice and the propensity to blame the victim of inequality. The reproduction of social patterns of inequality inflicted on individual life courses is at the heart of conceptualizing the collective and moral nature of society.

The use of the life-course perspective can also prevent the concept of "society" becoming dehumanized. Giddens' term "structuration" expresses the way in which powerful patterns of social behaviour form themselves through historical time. A parallel can be drawn between this concept and that of Elias in his long-term strands of interconnection running through historical societies, a process he calls "interweaving" or "figurations". Both concepts summarize a long-term unfolding process which involves both individual and collective action in ways that seek to avoid simplistic distinctions between free will and social determinism. My argument is that adding the concept of life course can strengthen these kinds of theories. It provides a link between key social processes: historical development and change, the patterns of cohort and generation, the experiences and choices of individuals, and their personal development. Embedded in the idea of life course is the sequence of cohorts, each with its own specific experience and contribution to history; our society did not begin and will not end with ourselves. The idea of life course directs our attention to the fact that social life entails mutual collective responsibility through time. The circumstances in which a cohort is able to exercise "choice" is partly inherited from previous cohorts and will have consequences for the "choices" of succeeding cohorts. The moral logic of this position is therefore that we have to act socially as trustees of the world for following generations.

The life course: its sociological and moral significance

On a personal level, such a life-course perspective enables me to make sense of the links between my grandparents' (born in the 1880s) commitment to Methodism, my parents' (born 1910 and 1911) commitment to pacifism and radical socialism, my own commitment (born 1947) to green and Third World issues, my son's (born 1972) taking-up of anti-racist causes and my daughter's (born 1969) participation in Methodist self-help groups. This perspective also gives me confidence that the struggles my grandchildren (born 1989 and 1990) will take up will not be between their and my generation but against the forms of structured dependence prevalent in their time. Importantly, these concepts, used carefully, can be useful in a cross-cultural context and aid an understanding of the plurality of cultures. It helps us make sense of the relatively care-free lives of young Nuer girls as described by Evans-Pritchard (1965); assists in making the inferior status of Tiwi bachelors more intelligible (Hart & Pilling 1960); gives insight into why widowhood is so problematic in India (Srinivas 1978, Caplan 1985) and why in our industrial society the representatives of capital are so concerned about the redistributive consequences of pension schemes.

On a theoretical level the life-course perspective can make a useful contribution to resolving problems in social theory revolving around the "society"/"individual" dichotomy. It offers one method of escaping the chicken and egg dilemma of conceptualizing either society or the individual as taking analytical priority. The idea of the life course avoids reifying the individual into an ideal-typical moral unit which alone has value and reality. It does this by seeing particular people as historically changing personalities with a life-time's career of

191

changing and developing roles and status. Similarly from the life-course perspective the concept "society" is not reified into an inanimate machine but encompasses people's humanity by seeing their current life course as structuring but not determining their subsequent lives. Society is seen from this perspective as the collective experience, knowledge, wisdom and prejudices of people throughout their life courses that shapes their knowledge and power in the present. It is the interweaving of life courses through time that relieves us of the necessity of regarding either the individual or society as fixed starting points in explaining patterns of inequality.

It is possible to argue that sociology normally constructs "the individual" as a body at a particular place and time. This conception of the individual becomes expressed through tables of incomes or voting intentions where individuals in this sense are counted up according to specified attributes of that body at a particular time and place. For considerations of equity and a proper sociology the conception of "the individual" should be that of a complete life course. Jones in this context has an identity of meaning with Jones's life – count no man happy till he is dead, as the Greeks put it. This conception is common in everyday culture, and more common in non-Western small-scale culture. It should be taken up into sociology as an alternative construction of "the individual" for theory and research. Once this step is taken, the moral claims of old people are part of the claims by "the individual/person as a whole" upon the prevailing sense of what is just. Further, such a conception circumvents previous sociological theories of inequality whose limitations stem from "snapshot" positions that theorize about hypothesized units at fixed points of time, when what is needed are theories and research comparing life courses. This I believe is a major original insight with which a human sociology can be built.

Such an approach allows further criticism of conventional sociological theories of inequality for not clearly specifying the elements that are unequal. Most theories of inequality treat variously offices/occupations, roles/individual agents/social locations, at an instant or over a short period as units of analysis. Most beneficially, they should look at the whole person, a process that involves taking a life-course perspective. For theories of inequality that start from materialist accounts, including theories of exploitation, the balance of returns from labour over the life course should be the central focus.

Imagine a society where every individual takes the same life-course progress up an extremely steep hierarchy of more and more privileged status and eventually dies at the top having been born at the bottom. Is this an equal society? The problem comes with the steepness of the hierarchy and the differential power relations. The most egalitarian societies are those societies in which every member comes, over the life course, to hold a position of high status. These are frequently small-scale hunting and gathering societies. Moreover, the smallness of scale enables people to be treated as full personalities with life histories rather than structured by single attributes. These societies are not only small scale but their differentials of power, while they do exist, are not those of modern capitalism. A society experiencing the introduction of steep hierarchies and large power differentials would see inequalities becoming fossilized, and over time it would become clear that the reproduction of stratification processes had set in. This happened to many societies through colonialism.

The most important theme of this book is that the life course constitutes a sociological and a moral unit. The original perspective elaborated through this book is that people should be understood in terms of their life course – as producer and as product of a life course. That which people have become in the present, and that potential they have for the future, is a creation of their life course. Thus from a sociological perspective, issues of inequality should be seen as a life-course phenomenon. People should not be divided up and thought about by individual characteristics of age or gender or class or race or disability or other single strands of identity. They should be looked at as the current expression of a life course that obviously includes a wide range of attributes each and all of which impact on the course of that life. Similar life-course principles should apply to moral attributions. Looking at old people as an age strata that is waiting to die, a functionless remnant of people who are without status or significance, is demeaning, unnecessary and unhelpful and can be linked to the extreme individualism of our society. It can be combated by paying attention to the moral worth of the total life course and not merely one part of it. People make an enormous variety of contributions to and demands on society through their life course and the society in which we now live is the concrete product of that collection of life courses. We live in the legacy of the past, that past significantly includes the life course of elderly people alive at the moment. Without their activities and achievements the world would be a different place. This idea is reflected in the rural wisdom of the need for each generation to protect the fertility of the soil – "Lime, lime and no manure make the fathers rich and the sons poor". Thus it is necessary for a proper insight into inequality in our society to review individual and collective contributions to the state of the world, past, present and future. The concept of life course is an essential tool for conceptualizing society as the product of the interweaving of all our experiences and actions. This life-course perspective can also give a more accurate and more positive moral evaluation of the position of old people. Reminiscence therapy is very helpful to many old people; they are given time and help to review their lives, to remember what they have done and achieved that can give them a sense of their own value in old age. Further, society at large should pause to listen to their stories, to know what they contributed to make society what it is today. Not only is the idea of life-course review of practical value to elderly people in understanding themselves but it is of significant importance in aiding us collectively to understand ourselves and our own society (Sherman & Webb 1994, Bornat 1993). Biography is one of the most popular forms of literature – the life stories of the great, the good and the notorious are widely read. Literature on old people as a social category is likely to be about victims, passive creatures to which things happen; whereas biographies of elderly people are more likely to be about heroes and heroines, or perhaps villains, but certainly people who are active and who contribute to making things happen.

The idea of life course also helps sort out the issues of old age, disability and death. Rather than old age taking its meaning from disability, particularly through the medicalization of old age, old age and death would take their rightful and meaningful place in the social passage of time; not as isolated events to be feared and hidden but as a fitting part of a meaningful and valued event called a life course. Disability rather is a feature of society which is structured in such a way as not to allow the abilities of many people to be fully developed. Mobility only becomes a problem when mobility is socially required. This argument becomes particularly acute when looking at the severely mentally handicapped and advanced dementia approaching on vegetative states. Issues of death and disability do come together in the discussion of euthanasia. From one view, voluntary euthanasia can be a meaningful coda to a worthwhile life course; to others there is the danger of the most powerless having their lives structured to an end to meet the needs of powerful others.

The Eskimo elders abandoned for the collective good (Simmons 1970) might be contrasted with the Tikopia young men launched on a one-way voyage into the ocean at equivalent times of scarcity (Firth 1957: 373-4). The issue here then is domination, it is domination which gives moral meaning to the event. Who is doing the structuring of others' lives such that they end them, the elder chiefs of Tikopia, the active Eskimo hunters, the consultant high priests of the medical profession or a fully satisfied liberated elder of an equalitarian Utopia?

The two fashionable intellectual trends of the 1980s were the libertarian free-market views of the new right that were politically ascendant, and the postmodern approaches to philosophy that have become ascendant in the intellectual and academic communities. They both have a bizarre inability to come to terms with concrete issues of inequality. The new right argue that there is an identity between equality and sameness – that an equal society is impossible because we are not all the same but are naturally different. The postmodern view of the world is that order and regularity are breaking down into a plurality of lifestyles that are incommensurable, any cultural value scheme is as good as the next. From a "postmodern" position the issue of inequality ultimately becomes irrelevant, for who can judge whose account of disadvantage is closer to the truth, whose vision of a better society is more plausible. However, the postmodern perspective gives the lie to the idea that equality means the elimination of difference. On the contrary, true progressive visions celebrate difference, welcome variety and do not accept that the discipline of the market is any more tolerant of cultural diversity than other institutions. The problem is not differentiation; it is domination. However, postmodern approaches do not seem to subject their own relativistic and pluralistic assumptions to the same critical analyses they apply to modernist meta-narratives. We cannot do away with moral philosophy completely. Any social science worth its salt, and able to influence the world at large, has to have a value position and it is better that these are made explicit and examined.

Despite the scepticism concerning "meta-narratives" (Lyotard 1984) in much current sociology/anthropology there is a need for a unified theory of inequality so that we can be more than passive spectators to the massive social changes currently taking place. This theory needs to be global and to emphasize social processes rather than proliferating categories of disadvantage. It should link cultural

195

and material processes, and provide an aid to understanding historically specific situations without being prescriptive or over-deterministic. All existing theories fail to meet this specification adequately. Systematically thinking through inequality in old age provides new insights appropriate for constructing a more general theory of social inequality. In particular, by demanding that theories encompass the whole life course, including sections such as old age that have been regarded as peripheral, and identifying inequality as a relationship of situated life courses, a major reconceptualization of inequality can emerge.

Thus the concluding argument of this book is that ageism cannot be challenged by itself. What has to be understood, revealed and rolled back are the processes of exploitation and hegemony by which not only ageism but sexism and racism are perpetuated and expanded. The generation of a non-exploitative moral economy and the generation of the cultural practices of freedom and creativity, like all good basic humanistic values, have to be strived for. A society that strives for those values will in the long run diminish all inequalities. Furthermore, this has to be accompanied by a sense of people in history. By this I mean it is, in the long run, not beneficial or productive to work for the betterment of merely one's own cohort when we are old, or even to strive for better treatment of elders as an age strata. What is really required is a weakening of the power of the processes of domination. It is by people gaining a sense of themselves as having a place in the continuity of human history that the elderly can take pride of place as the link between past and living generations. Elderly people can come to be valued as symbols of the continuity of generations, provided that continuity is valued. The idea of old people as at the fag end of their lives, parasiting on the rest of society, can be defeated, provided we have a collective sense of our own history and our own destiny. The ecological necessity to cherish the earth, its resources and environment for future generations should lead to a sense of historical continuity and responsibility which in turn will lead to a revaluation of older people in our society. The elderly are moral pioneers (Silverman 1987b); new settlers moving into the virgin territories of longevity and seeking there the full potential of a meaningful long life. It is unlikely that others, particularly those firmly attached to the well-trodden paths of the traditional life course, will be able to map out meaningful ways of living to these pioneers. What needs to happen is that we must collectively strive to build a community of values that does not devalue and restrict people on the basis of age criteria. Further, we need to strive for an institutional structure and a division of social labour that rather than exploiting people (including older people) offers the possibility of equal and mutually beneficial exchange between generations. In these circumstances a proper and effective moral revaluation of later years is likely to emerge.

Bibliography

Abercrombie, N. & A. Warde 1988. *Contemporary British society*. Cambridge: Polity.

Achenbaum, A. W. 1983. *Shades of gray: old age, American values, and federal policies since 1920*. Boston: Little, Brown.

Amoss, P. T. & S. Harrell 1981. *Other ways of growing old*. Stanford Calif.: Stanford University Press.

Anderson, B. 1991. *Imagined communities*, 2nd edn. New York: Verso.

Antonucci, T. & J. Jackson 1989. Successful ageing and life course reciprocity. In *Human ageing and later life: multidisciplinary perspectives*, A. M. Warnes (ed.), 83–95. London: Edward Arnold.

Anwar, M. 1979. *The myth of the return: Pakistanis in Britain*. London: Heinemann.

Arber, S. 1989. Class and the elderly. *Social Studies Review* **4**(3), 90–95.

Arber, S. & G. N. Gilbert 1989. Transitions in caring: gender, life course, and the care of the elderly. In *Becoming and being old: sociological approaches to later life*, W. Bytheway (ed.), 72–92. London: Sage.

Arber, S., G. N. Gilbert, M. Evandrou 1988. Gender, household composition and receipt of domiciliary services by elderly disabled people. *Journal of Social Policy* **17**, 153–75.

Arber, S. & J. Ginn 1990. The meaning of informal care: gender and the contribution of elderly people. *Ageing and Society* **10**, 429–54.

Arber, S. & J. Ginn 1991. *Gender and later life*. London: Sage.

Arensberg, C. M. & S. T. Kimball 1940. *Family and community in Ireland*. Gloucester, Mass.: Peter Smith.

Askham, J., L. Henshaw, M. Tarpey 1993. Policies and perceptions of identity, service needs of elderly people from black and minority ethnic backgrounds. In *Ageing, independence and the life course*, S. Arber & M. Evandrou (eds), 169–85. London: Jessica Kingsley.

Bailey, F. G. 1971. The peasant view of the bad life. In *Peasants and peasant societies*, T. Shanin (ed.), 299–321. Harmondsworth: Penguin.

Baltes, P. B. & M. M. Baltes 1990. *Successful aging: perspectives from the behavioural sciences.* Cambridge: Cambridge University Press.

Baltes, P. B., K. U. Mayer, H. Helmchen, E. Steinhagen-Thiessen 1993. The Berlin Aging Study. *Ageing and Society.* Special Issue **13**(4).

Banton, M. 1983. *Racial and ethnic competition.* Cambridge: Cambridge University Press.

Banton, M. 1987. *Racial theories.* Cambridge: Cambridge University Press.

Barth, F. 1969. *Ethnic groups and boundaries.* London: Allen & Unwin.

Bauman, Z. 1992. *Mortality, immortality, and other life strategies.* Cambridge: Polity.

Bengston, V. 1990. Plenary address to the 2nd International Conference on the Adult Lifecourse, Leeuwenhorst, Netherlands (July 1990).

Bernardi, B. 1985. *Age class systems: social institutions and polities based on age.* Cambridge: Cambridge University Press.

Berndt, C. H. & R. M. Berndt 1983. *The Aboriginal Australians: the first pioneers*, 2nd edn. Victoria, Australia: Pitman.

Biggs, S. 1993. *Understanding ageing: images, attitudes and professional practice.* Buckingham: Open University Press.

Black, M. 1973. Belief systems. In *Handbook of social and cultural anthropology*, J. J. Honigman (ed.), chap. 12. Chicago: Rand MacNally.

Blaikie, A. & J. Mcnicol 1986. Towards an anatomy of ageism: society, social policy and the elderly between the wars. In *Dependency and interdependency in old age*, C. Phillipson, M. Bernard, P. Y. Strang (eds), 95–104. London: Croom Helm.

Blakemore, K. & M. Boneham 1994. *Age, race and ethnicity.* Buckingham: Open University Press.

Blau, P. 1964. *Exchange and power in social life.* New York: Wiley.

Bloch, M. 1971. *Placing the dead: tombs, ancestral villages and kinship organisation in Madagascar.* London: Seminar Press.

Bloch, M. 1989. *Ritual, history and power.* London: Athlone Press.

Bodely, J. H. 1983. *Anthropology and contemporary human problems*, 2nd edn. Mountain View, Calif.: Mayfield.

Bond, J. & P. Coleman (eds) 1990. *Ageing in society.* London: Sage.

Bornat, J. 1993. Oral history as a social movement: reminiscence and older people. In *Ageing and later life*, J. Johnson & R. Salter (eds), 280–87. London: Sage.

Boserup, E. 1970. *Women's role in economic development.* London: Allen & Unwin.

Briggs, R. 1990. Biological ageing. In *Ageing in society*, J. Bond & P. Coleman (eds), chap. 3. London: Sage.

Brodkin, S. K. 1989. Towards a unified theory of class, race, and gender. *American Ethnologist* **16**, 534–50.

Bromley, D. B. 1988. *Human ageing: an introduction to gerontology.* London: Penguin.

Bytheway, W. (ed.) 1989. *Becoming and being old: sociological approaches to later life.* London: Sage.

Bytheway, W. 1995. *Ageism.* Buckingham: Open University Press.

Caplan, P. 1985. *Class and gender in India.* London: Tavistock.

Caplovitz, D. 1963. *The poor pay more*. New York: The Free Press.
Carnegie inquiry into the Third Age, 1993. *Life, work and livelihood in the Third Age*. Dunfermline, Scotland: Carnegie United Kingdom Trust.
Central Statistical Office 1992. *Family spending: report on the 1991 family expenditure survey*. London: HMSO.
Chagnon, N. 1977. *The Yanamamo*. New York: Holt, Rinehart & Winston.
Clark, D. (ed.) 1993. *The sociology of death*. Oxford: Blackwell.
Clarke, E. 1957. *My mother who fathered me*. London: Allen & Unwin.
Cole, T. R. 1992. *The journey of life: a cultural history of aging in America*. Cambridge: Cambridge University Press.
Cole, T. R. 1993. *Voices and visions of ageing: toward a critical gerontology*. New York: Springer.
Coleman, P. G. 1991. Ageing and life history: the meaning of reminiscence in late life. In *Life and work history analyses*, S. Dex (ed.), 120–43. London: Routledge.
Comfort, A. 1977. *A good age*. London: Pan Book.
Cool, B. E. 1987. The effects of social class and ethnicity on the aging process. In *The elderly as modern pioneers*, P. Silverman (ed.), 263–82. Bloomington, Ind.: Indiana University Press.
Corbridge, S. 1986. *Capitalist world development: a critique of radical development geography*. Basingstoke: Macmillan.
Cowen, T. & D. Parfit 1992. Against the social discount rate. In *Justice between age groups and generations*, P. Laslett & J. S. Fishkin (eds), 144–61. New Haven, Conn.: Yale University Press.
Cowgill, D. O. & L. D. Holmes 1972. *Aging and modernisation*. New York: Appleton Century.
Cribier, F. 1989. Changes in life course and retirement in recent years: the example of two cohorts of Parisians. In *Workers versus pensioners*, P. Johnson, C. Conrad, D. Thomson (eds), 181–201. Manchester: Manchester University Press in association with the Centre for Economic Policy Research.
Crompton, R. & K. Sanderson 1990. *Gendered jobs and social change*. London: Unwin Hyman.
Cumming, E. & W. Henry 1961. *Growing old: the process of disengagement*. New York: Basic Books.
Czechoslovak Demographic Society 1989. Proceedings of the International Population Conference. Ageing of population in developed countries. In *Acta Demographica* **9**.
Dahlberg, F. 1981. *Woman the gatherer*. New Haven, Conn.: Yale University Press.
De Bary, W. T., A. L. Bashar, R. N. Dandekar 1958. *Sources of Indian tradition*. New York: Columbia University Press.
de Beauvoir, S. 1972. *Old age*. London: André Deutsch and Weidenfeld & Nicolson.
Deere, C. D., J. Humphries, M. Leon de Leal 1982. Class and historical analysis for the study of women and social change. In *Women's roles and population trends in the Third World*, R. Anker, M. Buvinic, N. M. Youssef (eds), 87–116. London: Croom Helm.

Dex, S. (ed.) 1991. *Life and work history analyses*. London: Routledge.

Dickenson, D. & M. Johnson (eds) 1993. *Death, dying and bereavement*. London: Sage.

Donner, F. 1982. *Shabono*. London: Paladin Books.

Douglas, M. (ed.) 1973. *Rules and meanings*. Harmondsworth: Penguin.

Dragadze, T. 1990. The notion of adulthood in rural Soviet Georgian society. In *Anthropology and the riddle of the sphinx*, P. Spenser (ed.), 89–101. London: Routledge.

Dressel, P. L. 1991. Gender, race and class: beyond the feminization of poverty in later life. In *Critical perspectives on aging: the political and moral economy of growing old*, M. Minkler & C. Estes (eds), 245–52. Amityville, New York: Baywood.

Durkheim, E. & M. Mauss 1963. *Primitive classification*. London: Cohen & West.

Eisenstadt, S. N. 1956. *From generation to generation*. London: Collier-Macmillan.

Elias, N. 1978. *What is sociology?* London: Hutchinson.

Elias, N. 1982. *The civilising process*. Oxford: Blackwell.

Elias, N. 1985. *The loneliness of dying*. Oxford: Blackwell.

Emmanuel, A. 1972. *Unequal exchange*. London: Monthly Review Press.

Engels, F. (1884, 1942) 1972. *The origin of the family, private property, and the state*, trans. and ed. E. Leacock & A. West. London: Lawrence & Wishart.

Erickson, E. 1963. *Childhood and society*, 2nd edn. New York: Norton.

Erickson, E. 1982. *The life cycle completed: a review*. New York: Norton.

Ermisch, J. 1989. Welfare, age, and generation: demographic change and intergenerational transfers in industrialised countries. In *Workers versus pensioners: intergenerational justice in an ageing world*, P. Johnson, C. Conrad, D. Thomson (eds), 17–33. Manchester: Manchester University Press in association with the Centre for Economic Policy Research.

Estes, C. L. 1979. *The aging enterprise*. San Francisco: Josey-Bass.

Estes, C. L., L. E. Gerard, J. Sprague-Zones, J. H. Swan 1984. *Political economy, health, and aging*. Boston: Little, Brown.

Estes, C. L. & M. Minkler 1984. *Readings in the political economy of aging*. Farmingdale, New York: Baywood.

Estes, C. L., J. H. Swan, and associates 1993. *The long-term care crisis: elders trapped in the no-care zone*. Newbury Park, Calif.: Sage.

Evandrou, M. & C. Victor 1989. Differentiation in later life: social class and housing tenure cleavages. In *Becoming and being old: sociological approaches to later life*, W. Bytheway (ed.), 105–20. London: Sage.

Evans-Pritchard, E. E. 1940. *The Nuer: a description of the modes of livelihood and political institutions of a Nilotic people*. Oxford: Oxford University Press.

Evans-Pritchard, E. E. 1965. *The position of women in primitive societies and other essays in social anthropology*. London: Faber & Faber.

Family Expenditure Survey 1985, 1988, 1992 (accessed through Manchester University Computing Centre Data Archive).

Fanon, F. 1967. *The wretched of the earth*. Harmondsworth: Penguin.

Fanon, F. 1968. *Black masks, white faces*. London: Pluto.

Farb, P. 1969. *Man's rise to civilisation as shown by the Indians of North America from primeval times to the coming of the industrial state.* London: Martin Secker & Warburg.

Featherstone, M. 1982. The body in consumer culture. *Theory, Culture, and Society* **1**, 18–33.

Featherstone, M. & M. Hepworth 1989. Ageing and old age: reflections on the postmodern life course. In *Becoming and being old: sociological approaches to later life,* W. Bytheway (ed.), 143–57. London: Sage.

Fennell, G. 1986. Structured dependency revisited. In *Dependency and interdependency in old age,* C. Phillipson, M. Bernard, P. Strang (eds), 54–68. Beckenham, Kent: Croom Helm.

Fennell, G., C. Phillipson, H. Evers 1988. *The sociology of old age.* Milton Keynes, England: Open University Press.

Finch, J. 1987. Family obligations and the life course. In *Rethinking the life cycle,* A. Bryman, B. Bytheway, P. Allat, T. Keil (eds), 155–69. Basingstoke: Macmillan.

Finch, J. 1989. *Family obligations and social change.* Cambridge: Polity.

Finch, J. & J. Mason 1990. Divorce, remarriage and family obligations. *The Sociological Review* **38**, 219–46.

Firth, R. 1957. *We, the Tikopia,* 2nd edn. Boston: Beacon Press.

Foner, N. 1976a. Jamaicans. In *Between two cultures,* J. L. Watson (ed.), 120–50. Oxford: Blackwell.

Foner, N. 1976b. Women, work, and migration: Jamaicans in London. *New Community* **5**, 85–98.

Foner, N. 1984. *Age in conflict: a cross-cultural perspective on inequality between old and young.* New York: Columbia Press.

Frake, C. 1962. The ethnographic study of cognitive systems. In *Anthropology and human behaviour,* T. Gladwin & W. C. Sturtevant (eds), 72–85. Washington: Anthropological Society of Washington.

Frank, A. G. 1967. *Capitalism and underdevelopment in Latin America.* London: Monthly Review Press.

Friedan, B. 1993. *The fountain of age.* London: Vintage.

General Household Survey 1987, 1991/2 (accessed through Manchester University Computing Centre Data Archive).

Giddens, A. 1984. *The constitution of society.* Cambridge: Polity.

Giddens, A. 1991. *Modernity and self-identity.* Cambridge: Polity.

Gilroy, P. 1987. *There ain't no black in the Union Jack.* London: Hutchinson.

Gingold, R. 1992. *Successful ageing.* Melbourne: Oxford University Press.

Glaser, B. & A. Strauss 1965. *The awareness of dying.* Chicago: Aldine.

Goldthorpe, J. E. 1975. *The sociology of the Third World: disparity and involvement.* Cambridge: Cambridge University Press.

Goodenough, W. C. 1964. *Explorations in cultural anthropology.* New York: McGraw Hill.

Goodenough, W. C. 1968. Componential analysis. In *Encyclopedia of the social sciences.* New York: Crowell, Collier & MacMillan.

Goody, J. 1990. *The Oriental, the ancient and the primitive: systems of marriage and the family in the pre-industrial societies of Eurasia.* Cambridge: Cambridge University Press.

Gramsci, A. 1971. *Selections from the prison notebooks of Antonio Gramsci*, Q. Hoare & G. Nowell Smith (eds). London: Lawrence & Wishart.

Greer, Germaine 1993. Youthism. Channel 4, 16 October.

Grillis, J. R. 1987. The case against chronologization; changes in the Anglo-American life cycle 1600 to the present. *Ethnologia Europaea* **17**, 97–106.

Guillemard, A-M. 1989. The trend towards early labour force withdrawal and reorganisation of the life course: a cross-national analysis. In *Workers versus pensioners*, P. Johnson, C. Conrad, D. Thomson (eds), 163–80. Manchester: Manchester University Press in association with the Centre for Economic Policy Research.

Guillemard, A-M. 1990. Re-organising the transition from work to retirement in an international perspective: is chronological age still the major criterion determining the definitive exit? Paper presented to the International Sociological Association Conference, Madrid 1990.

Habermas, J. 1971. *Towards a rational society*. London: Heinemann.

Habermas, J. 1984. *The theory of communicative action*. London: Heinemann.

Hall, S. & T. Jefferson (eds) 1976. *Resistance through rituals: youth subcultures in post-war Britain*. London: Hutchinson.

Hamnett, C. 1989. Consumption and class in contemporary Britain. In *The changing social structure*, C. Hamnett, L. McDowell, P. Sarre (eds), 199–243. London: Sage.

Hareven, T. K. 1982. *Family time and industrial time*. Cambridge: Cambridge University Press.

Harris, C. 1987. The individual and society: a process approach. In *Rethinking the life cycle*, A. Bryman, W. Bytheway, P. Allatt, T. Keil (eds), chap. 1. Basingstoke: Macmillan.

Harris, C. C. 1990. *Kinship*. Milton Keynes, England: Open University Press.

Hart, C. W. M. & A. R. Pilling 1960. *The Tiwi of North Australia*. New York: Holt, Rinehart & Winston.

Hazan, H. 1994. *Old age: Constructions and deconstructions*. Cambridge: Cambridge University Press.

Hebdige, D. 1979. *Subculture: the meaning of style*. London: Methuen.

Hedstrom, P. & S. Ringen 1987. Age and income in contemporary society: a research note. *Journal of Social Policy* **16**, 227–39.

Hendricks, J. & C. A. Leedham 1991. Dependency or empowerment? Toward a moral and political economy of aging. In *Critical perspectives on aging: the political and moral economy of growing old*, M. Minkler & C. Estes (eds), 51–66. Amityville, New York: Baywood.

Henwood, M. 1990. No sense of urgency: age discrimination in health care. In *Age: the unrecognised discrimination*, E. McEwen (ed.), 43–57. London: Age Concern England.

Hepworth, M. 1987. The mid-life phase. In *Social change and the life course*, G. Cohen (ed.), 134–55. London: Tavistock.

Hepworth, M. & M. Featherstone 1982. *Surviving middle age*. Oxford: Blackwell.

Hilgard, S. R. 1979. *Introduction to psychology*. London: Harcourt-Brace.

Hilton, I. 1993. Profile: Germaine Greer – another age another rage. *Independent*, 17 October.

Hobsbawm, E. 1992. *Nations and nationalism since 1780*, 2nd edn. Cambridge: Cambridge University Press.

Hockey, J. & A. James 1993. Growing up and growing old: a discussion of ageing and dependency in the life course. *Generations Review* 3(4), 2–4.

Hooyman, N. & H. A. Kiyak 1988. *Social gerontology*. Boston: Allyn & Bacon.

Horowitz, M. M. 1967. *Morne paysan*. New York: Holt, Rinehart & Winston.

Horowitz, M. M. (ed.) 1971. *Peoples and cultures of the Caribbean*. New York: Natural History Press.

Hugman, R. 1994. *Ageing and the care of older people in Europe*. Basingstoke: Macmillan.

Hymes, D. 1964. *Language in culture and society*. New York: Harper & Row.

Ikels, C., K. Diskerson-Putman, J. Draper, C. Fry, A. Glascock, H. Harpending 1992. Perceptions of the adult life course: a cross-cultural analysis. *Ageing and Society* 12(1), 49–84.

Imhof, A. E. 1987. Planning a full-size life career: consequences of the increase in the length and certainty of our life spans over the last 300 years. *Ethnologia Europaea* 17(1), 5–23.

Johnson, C. L. 1988a. *Ex familia – grandparents, parents, and children adjust to divorce*. New Brunswick, New Jersey: Rutgers University Press.

Johnson, C. L. 1988b. Postdivorce reorganization of relationships between divorcing children and their parents. *Journal of Marriage and the Family* 50(1), 221–31.

Johnson, C. L., L. Klee, C. Schmidt 1988. Conceptions of parentage and kinship among children of divorce. *American Anthropologist* 90(1), 136–44.

Johnson, M. 1978. That was your life: a biographical approach to later life. In *An ageing population*, V. Carver & P. Liddiard (eds), 99–113. Sevenoaks, England: Open University/ Hodder & Stoughton.

Johnson, M. 1993. Generational relations under review. In *Uniting generations: studies in conflict and co-operation*, D.Hobman (ed.), 12–29. London: Age Concern England.

Johnson, P. 1985. *The economics of old age in Britain: a long-run view 1881–1981*. Discussion paper no. 47. London: Centre for Economic Policy Research.

Johnson, P., C. Conrad, D. Thomson (eds) 1989. *Workers versus pensioners: intergenerational justice in an ageing world*. Manchester: Manchester University Press in association with the Centre for Economic Policy Research.

Johnson, P. & J. Falkingham, 1992. *Ageing and economic welfare*. London: Sage.

Joshi, H. (ed.) 1989. *The changing population of Britain*. Oxford: Blackwell.

Karn, V. A. 1977. *Retiring to the seaside*. London: Routledge & Kegan Paul.

Khan, V. S. 1976. Pakistani women in Britain. *New Community* 5, 99–103.

Kirk, H. 1992. Geriatric medicine and the categorisation of old age – the historical linkage. *Ageing and Society* 12, 484–97.

Kohli, M. 1986. The world we forgot: a historical review of the life course. In *Later life: the social psychology of aging*, V. W. Marshall (ed.), 271–303. London: Sage.

Kohli, M. 1990. Plenary address to the 2nd International Conference on the Adult Lifecourse, Leeuwenhorst, Netherlands (July 1990).

Kohli, M. 1991. Retirement and the moral economy: an historical interpretation of the German case. In *Critical perspectives on aging: the political and moral economy of growing old*, M. Minkler & C. Estes (eds), 273–92. Amityville, New York: Baywood.

Kohli, M., M. Rein, A-M. Guillemard, H. Van Gunstern (eds) 1992. *Time for retirement: comparative studies on early exit for the labour force.* Cambridge: Cambridge University Press.

Laczko, F. & C. Phillipson 1991. *Changing work and retirement.* Milton Keynes, England: Open University Press.

La Fontaine, J. S. 1978. *Sex and age as principles of social differentiation.* ASA Monograph 17. London: Academic Press.

La Fontaine, J. S. 1985. *Initiation: ritual drama and secret knowledge across the world.* Harmondsworth: Penguin.

Laslett, P. 1968. *The world we have lost.* London: Methuen.

Laslett, P. 1989. *A fresh map of life: the emergence of the Third Age.* London: Weidenfeld & Nicolson.

Laslett, P. 1992. Is there a generational contract? In *Justice between age groups and generations*, P. Laslett & J. S. Fishkin (eds), 24–47. New Haven, Conn.: Yale University Press.

Laslett, P. & J. S. Fishkin (eds) 1992. *Justice between age groups and generations.* New Haven, Conn.: Yale University Press.

Laslett, P. & R. Wall 1972. *Household and family in past times.* Cambridge: Cambridge University Press.

Lee, R. 1979. *The !Kung San: men, women and work in a foraging society.* Cambridge: Cambridge University Press.

Lee, R. B. & I. DeVore 1968. *Man the hunter.* Chicago: Aldine.

Letwin, W. (ed.) 1983. *Against equality.* London: Macmillan.

Lévi-Strauss, C. 1963. *Structural anthropology.* New York: Basic Books.

Lévi-Strauss, C. 1969. *The elementary structures of kinship.* London: Eyre & Spottiswoode.

Lévi-Strauss, C. 1970. *The raw and the cooked*, trans. J. & D. Weightman. London: Cape.

Lizot, J. 1985. *Tales of the Yanomami.* Cambridge: Cambridge University Press.

Lukes, S. 1974. *Power, a radical view.* London: Macmillan.

Lyotard, J-F. 1984. *The postmodern condition: a report on knowledge.* Minneapolis, Minn.: University of Minnesota Press.

McDowell, L., P. Sarre, C. Hamnett 1989. *Divided nation: social and cultural change in Britain.* London: Hodder & Stoughton.

McEwen, E. (ed.) 1990. *Age: The unrecognised discrimination.* London: Age Concern England.

McNay, L. 1992. *Foucault and feminism.* Cambridge: Polity.

Marshall, T. H. 1950. *Citizenship and social class and other essays.* Cambridge: Cambridge University Press.

Marshall, V. 1981. Toleration of ageing: sociological theory and social response to population ageing. Proceedings of the IXth International

Conference of Social Gerontology. Paris: International Centre of Social Gerontology.

Mayer, K. U. & M. Wagner 1993. Socio-economic resources and differential ageing. *Ageing and Society* **13**, 517–50.

Mayer, P. J. 1987. Biological theories of aging. In *The elderly as modern pioneers*, P. Silverman (ed.), 17–53. Bloomington, Ind.: Indiana University Press.

Meillassoux, C. 1983. The economic bases of demographic reproduction: from domestic mode of production to wage-earning. *Journal of Peasant Studies* **11**, 50–61.

Mellor, P. 1993. Death in high modernity: the contemporary presence and absence of death. In *The sociology of death*, D. Clark (ed.), 11–30. Oxford: Blackwell.

Mennell, S. J. 1977. "Individual" action and its "social" consequences in the work of Elias. In *Human figurations*, P. R. Gleichmann, J. Goudsblom, H. Korte (eds), 99–109. Amsterdam: Amsterdams Sociologisch Tijdschrift.

Meyer, J. W. 1988. Levels of analysis: the life course as a cultural construction. In *Social structures human lives, vol. 1 (Social change and the life course)*, M. W. Riley, B. J. Huber, B. Beth (eds), 49–62. Newbury Park, Calif. and London: Sage.

Midwinter, E. 1991. *The British Gas report on attitudes to ageing.* London: British Gas.

Midwinter, E. & S. Tester 1987. *Polls apart? Older voters at the 1987 election.* London: Centre for Policy of Ageing.

Miles, R. 1982. *Racism and migrant labour.* London: Routledge & Kegan Paul.

Mills, C. W. (1959) 1970. *The sociological imagination.* Harmondsworth: Penguin.

Mingione, E. 1981. *Social conflict and the city.* Oxford: Blackwell.

Minios, G. 1989. *History of old age: from antiquity to the Renaissance*, trans. S. H. Tenison. Cambridge: Polity.

Minkler, M. 1984. Blaming the aged victim: the politics of retrenchment in times of fiscal conservatism. In *Readings in the political economy of aging*, C. L. Estes & M. Minkler (eds), 254–69. Farmingdale, New York: Baywood.

Minkler, M. 1991. 'Generational equity' and the new victim blaming. In *Critical perspectives on aging: the political and moral economy of growing old*, M. Minkler & C. Estes (eds), 67–80. Amityville, New York: Baywood.

Minkler, M. & T. R. Cole 1991. Political and moral economy: not such strange bedfellows. In *Critical perspectives on aging: the political and moral economy of growing old*, M. Minkler & C. Estes (eds), 37–49. Amityville, New York: Baywood.

Minkler, M. & C. Estes (eds) 1991. *Critical perspectives on aging: the political and moral economy of growing old.* Amityville, New York: Baywood.

Momsen, J. H. & J. Townsend 1987. *Geography of gender in the Third World.* London: Hutchinson.

Moody, H. R. 1992. *Ethics in an aging society.* Baltimore: The Johns Hopkins University Press.

Musgrove, F. & R. Middleton 1981. Rites of passages and the meaning of age in three contrasted social groups. *British Journal of Sociology* **32**(1), 39–55.

Myrdal, A. 1945. *Nation and family.* London: Kegan Paul, Trench, Trubner.

Nelson, D. W. 1982. Alternative images of old age as the bases for policy. In *Age or need: public policies for older people,* B. L. Neugarten (ed.), 144–5. Beverly Hills, Calif.: Sage.

Neugarten, B. L. 1982. *Age or need: public policies for older people.* Beverly Hills, Calif.: Sage.

O'Donnell, M. 1985. *Age and generation.* London: Tavistock.

Office of Population Census and Surveys 1991. *1991 Census. Preliminary report for England and Wales.* London: HMSO.

Office of Population Census and Surveys 1993a. *1991 Historical tables: Great Britain.* London: HMSO.

Office of Population Census and Surveys 1993b. *1991 Census report for Great Britain (part 1).* London: HMSO.

Office of Population Census and Surveys 1993c. *General household survey.* Series GHS 22. London: HMSO.

Office of Population Census and Surveys 1993d. *General household survey: people aged 65 and over.* Series GHS 22, suppl. A. London: HMSO.

Office of Population Census and Surveys 1993e. *Population Trends* **72,** 44–50. London: HMSO.

Ogburn, W. F. 1964. Technology and governmental change. In *Culture and social change,* O. D. Duncan (ed.), 131–43. Chicago: University of Chicago Press.

Ortner, S. B. 1974. Is female to male as nature is to culture? In *Woman, culture and society,* M. Z. Rosaldo & L. Lamphere (eds), 67–88. Stanford: Stanford University Press.

Packard, V. 1963. *The waste makers.* Harmondsworth: Penguin.

Palmore, E. B. & V. Stone 1973. Predictors of longevity: a follow-up of the aged in Chapel Hill. *The Gerontologist* **13**(1), 88–90.

Pampel, F. C. & J. B. Williamson 1989. *Age, class, politics and the welfare state.* Cambridge: Cambridge University Press.

Philips, D. R., J. Vincent, S. Blacksell 1988. *Home from home: private residential accommodation for elderly people in Devon, England.* Sheffield: University of Sheffield Press and Community Care.

Phillipson, C. 1982. *Capitalism and the construction of old age.* London: Macmillan.

Phillipson, C., M. Bernard, P. Strang (eds) 1986. *Dependency and interdependency in old age.* Beckenham, Kent: Croom Helm.

Phillipson, C. & A. Walker 1986. *Ageing and social policy: a critical assessment.* Aldershot, England: Gower.

Polyani, K., C. Arensberg, H. Pearson (eds) 1957. *Trade and market in early empires.* Glencoe, Ill.: Free Press.

Pratt, H. J. 1976. *The gray lobby.* London: University of Chicago Press.

Preston, S. 1984. Children and the elderly in the United States. *Scientific American* **251,** 44–9.

Qureshi, H. & K. Simons 1987. Caring for elderly people. In *Give and take in families,* J. Brannen & G. Wilson (eds). London: Allen & Unwin.

Qureshi, H. & A. Walker 1989. *The caring relationship: elderly people and their families.* Basingstoke: Macmillan.

Redclift, M. 1984. *Development and the environmental crisis*. London: Methuen.

Redclift, N. & E. Mingione 1985. *Beyond employment: household, gender, and subsistence*. Oxford: Blackwell.

Rex, J. & D. Mason 1986. *Theories of race and ethnic relations*. Cambridge: Cambridge University Press.

Riley, M. W. (ed.) 1979. *Aging from birth to death*, vol. 1 (*Interdisciplinary perspectives*). Boulder, Col.: Westview Press for the American Association for the Advancement of Science.

Riley, M. W. 1988. On the significance of age in sociology. In *Social structures and human lives*, M. W. Riley, B. J. Huber, B. B. Hess (eds), 24–45. Newbury Park, Calif.: Sage.

Riley, M. W., R. P. Abeles, M. S. Teitelbaum (eds) 1983. *Aging from birth to death*, vol. 2 (*Sociotemporal perspectives*). Boulder, Col.: Westview Press for the American Association for the Advancement of Science.

Riley, M. W., A. Foner, J. Waring 1988a. A sociology of age. In *Handbook of sociology*, H. J. Smelser (ed.). Newbury Park, Calif.: Sage.

Riley, M. W., B. J. Huber, B. B. Hess (eds) 1988b. *Social structures & human lives*, vol. 1 (*Social change and the life course*). Newbury Park, Calif. and London: Sage.

Ringer, B. B. & E. R. Lawless 1989. *Race-ethnicity and society*. London: Routledge.

Robertson, A. 1991. The politics of Alzheimer's disease: a case study in apocalyptic demography. In *Critical perspectives on aging: the political and moral economy of growing old*, M. Minkler & C. Estes (eds), 135–52. Amityville, New York: Baywood.

Rorty, R. 1994. Habermas and Lyotard. In *Polity reader in social theory*, 160–71. Cambridge: Polity.

Rousseau, J. J. (1762) 1968. *The social contract* (trans. M. Cranston). Harmondsworth: Penguin.

Rowntree, S. B. 1901. *Poverty – a study of town life*. London: Macmillan.

Rudinger, G. & H. Thomae 1990. The Bonn Longitudinal Study of Aging: coping, life adjustment and life satisfaction. In *Successful aging: perspectives from the behavioural sciences*, P. B. Baltes & M. M. Baltes (eds), 265–95. Cambridge: Cambridge University Press.

Sabat, S. & R. Harre 1992. The construction and deconstruction of self in Alzheimer's disease. *Ageing and Society* **12**, 443–62.

Sahlins, M. 1968. *Tribesmen*. Englewood Cliffs, New Jersey: Prentice-Hall.

Samuel, R. & P. Thompson 1990. *The myths we live by*. London: Routledge.

Sanday, P. R. 1981. *Female power and male dominance*. Cambridge: Cambridge University Press.

Sanderson, S. K. 1990. *Social evolutionism*. Oxford: Blackwell.

Sangree, W. H. 1965. The Bantu Tiriki of Western Kenya. In *Peoples of Africa*, J. Gibbs (ed.), 41–80. New York: Holt, Rinehart & Winston.

Sansom, B. 1978. Sex, age and social control in mobs of the Darwin hinterland. In *Sex and age as principles of social differentiation*, ASA Monograph 17. J. S. La Fontaine (ed.), 89–108. London: Academic Press.

Saunders, P. 1981. *Social theory and the urban question*. London: Hutchinson.

Sen, K. 1994. *Ageing: debates on demographic transition and social policy.* London: Zed Books.

Sharma, U. 1980. *Women, work, and property in North West India.* London: Tavistock.

Sharp, L. 1952. Steel axes for stone age Australians. In *Human problems in technological change,* E. Spicer (ed.), 69–90. New York: Russell Sage Foundation.

Sherman, E. and T. A. Webb 1994. The self as process in late-life reminiscence: spiritual attributes. *Ageing and Society* **14**, 255–67.

Silverman, P. 1987a. Comparative studies. In *The elderly as modern pioneers,* P. Silverman (ed.), 312–44. Bloomington, Ind.: Indiana University Press.

Silverman, P. (ed.) 1987b. *The elderly as modern pioneers.* Bloomington, Ind.: Indiana University Press.

Simmons, L. W. 1970. *The role of the aged in primitive society.* Hamden: Archon Books (reprint of 1945 Yale University Press edn.).

Smeeding, T. M. 1991. Mountains or molehills: just what's so bad about aging societies anyway? In *Macro–micro linkages in sociology,* J. Huber (ed.), 208–20. Newbury Park, Calif.: Sage.

Smith, A. D. 1981. *The ethnic revival.* Cambridge: Cambridge University Press.

Smith, J., I. Wallerstein, H-D. Evers (eds) 1984. *Households and the world economy.* Beverly Hills, Calif.: Sage.

Smith, M. F. 1954. *Baba of Karo: a woman of the Muslim Hausa.* London: Faber.

Social Trends, 1989 and 1994. London: HMSO.

Sontag, S. 1978. The double standard of ageing. In *An ageing population: a reader and source book,* V. Carver & P. Liddiard (eds), 72–8. Sevenoaks: Hodder & Stoughton/ Open University Press.

Spencer, P. 1965. *The Samburu: a study of gerontocracy in a nomadic tribe.* London: Routledge & Kegan Paul.

Spencer, P. 1990. The riddled course: theories of age and its transformations. In *Anthropology and the riddle of the sphinx,* P. Spencer (ed.), 1–34. London: Routledge.

Srinivas, M. N. 1978. *The changing position of Indian women.* Delhi: Oxford University Press.

Strathern, M. 1980. No nature, no culture: the Hagen case. In *Nature, culture and gender,* P. C. MacCormack & S. Marilyn (eds), 174–222. Cambridge: Cambridge University Press.

Sudnow, D. 1967. *Passing on: the social organisation of dying.* Englewood Cliffs, New Jersey: Prentice-Hall.

Tawney, R. H. (1931) 1964. *Equality.* London: Allen & Unwin.

Thane, P. 1989. Old age: burden or benefit. In *The changing population of Britain,* H. Joshi (ed.), 56–71. Oxford: Blackwell.

Thompson, E. P. 1968. *The making of the English working class.* Harmondsworth: Penguin.

Thompson, E. P. 1971. Moral economy of the English crowd in the 18th century. *Past and Present* **50**, 76–136.

Thompson, P., C. Itzin, M. Abendstern 1990. *I don't feel old: the experience of later life.* Oxford: Oxford University Press.

Townsend, P. 1957. *The family life of old people: an inquiry in East London.* London: Routledge & Kegan Paul.

Townsend, P. 1979. *Poverty in the United Kingdom, a survey of household resources and standards of living.* Harmondsworth: Penguin.

Townsend, P. 1986. Ageism and social policy. In *Ageing and social policy: a critical assessment,* C. Phillipson & A. Walker (eds), 15–44. Aldershot, England: Gower.

Turnball, C. 1983. *The Mbuti pygmies.* New York: Holt, Rinehart & Winston.

Turnball, C. 1984. *The forest people.* London: Triad/Paladin.

Turner, B. S. 1984. *The body and society: explorations in social theory.* Oxford: Blackwell.

Turner, B. S. 1986. *Equality.* London: Tavistock.

Turner, B. S. 1987. *Medical power and social knowledge.* London: Sage.

UN Demographic Year Book 1991.

Ungerson, C. 1987. *Policy is personal: sex, gender, and informal care.* London: Tavistock.

United Nations 1993. *The sex and age distribution of the world populations: the 1992 revision.* New York: United Nations Publications.

Valkovics, E. 1989. Population ageing in perspective: past and future trends. *Acta Demographia* **9**(1), 26–79.

Van Tassel, D. & P. Stearns 1986. *Old age in a bureaucratic society.* New York: Greenwood Press.

Victor, C. & M. Evandrou 1987. Does class matter in later life? In *Social gerontology: new directions,* S. di Gregorio (ed.), 252–67. London: Croom Helm.

Vincent, J. A. 1973a. St. Maurice. In *Debate and compromise,* F. G. Bailey (ed.), 200–18. Oxford: Blackwell.

Vincent, J. A. 1973b. *St. Maurice: an alpine community,* PhD thesis, African and Asian Studies, University of Sussex.

Vincent, J. A. 1987. Work and play in an alpine community. In *Who from their labours rest?,* M. Bouquet & M. Winter (eds), 105–19. Aldershot, England: Avebury.

Vincent, J. A. & Z. Mudrovcic 1992. Family circumstances of elderly people: Bosnia and Devon compared. The British Sociological Association Annual Conference. Canterbury: University of Kent.

Vincent, J. A. & Z. Mudrovcic 1993. Perceptions of elderly people and old age in Bosnia and Hercegovina. In *Ageing, independence and the life course,* S. Arber & M. Evandrou (eds), 91–103. London: Jessica Kingsley.

Walby, S. 1990. *Theorizing patriarchy.* Oxford: Blackwell.

Walker, A. 1980. The social creation of poverty and dependency in old age. *Journal of Social Policy* **9**, 49–75.

Walker, A. 1987. The social construction of dependency in old age. In *The state or the market,* M. Loney, R. Bocock, J. Clarke, A. Cochrane, P. Graham, M. Wilson (eds), 41–57. London: Sage.

Walker, A. 1990a. The economic 'burden' of ageing and the prospect of intergenerational conflict. *Ageing and Society* **10**, 377–96.

Walker, A. 1990b. The benefits of old age? Age discrimination and social security. In *Age: the unrecognised discrimination*, E. McEwen (ed.), 58–70. London: Age Concern England.

Walker, A. 1990c. Poverty and inequality in old age. In *Ageing society*, J. Bond & P. Coleman (eds), 229–49. London: Sage.

Walker, A. 1993. Whither the social contract? Intergenerational solidarity in income and employment. In *Uniting generations: studies in conflict and co-operation*, D. Hobman (ed.), 30–53. London: Age Concern England.

Wallerstein, I. 1974. *The modern world system*. New York: Academic Press.

Wallerstein, I. 1979. *The capitalist world economy*. Cambridge: Cambridge University Press.

Wallman, S. 1978. The boundaries of 'race': processes of ethnicity in England. *Man* **13**, 200–17.

Warnes, A. M. 1982. *Geographical perspectives on the elderly*. Chichester, England: John Wiley.

Warnes, A. M. 1987. The distribution of the elderly population of Great Britain. *Espace Populations Sociétés* **1**, 41–56.

Watcher, K. W., E. A. Hammel, P. Laslett 1978. *Statistical studies of historical social structure*. New York: Academic Press.

Weber, M. 1978. *Economy and society* [2 volumes], G. Roth & C. Wittich trans. and eds. Berkeley, Calif.: University of California Press.

Weissleder, W. (ed.) 1978. *The Nomadic alternative: modes and models of interaction in the African–Asian deserts and steppes*. The Hague: Mouton.

Wenger, C. 1984. *The supportive network: coping with old age*. London: Allen & Unwin.

Wenger, C. 1986. A longitudinal study of changes and adaptation in the support networks of Welsh elderly over 75. *Journal of Cross-Cultural Gerontology* **1**, 277–304.

Wenger, C. 1990. Change and adaptation in informal support networks of elderly people in Wales 1979–1987. *Journal of Aging Studies* **4**, 375–89.

White, L. A. 1959. *The evolution of culture*. New York: McGraw-Hill.

Williams, F. 1990. Race, gender, and class in the construction of social policy. The British Sociological Association Annual Conference. Guildford: University of Surrey.

Willis, P. 1977. *Learning to labour*. London: Saxon House.

Wilson, G. 1987. Women's work: the role of grandparents in intergenerational transfers. *The Sociological Review* **35**, 703–20.

Wilterdink, N. 1977. Norbert Elias's sociology of knowledge and its significance for the study of the sciences. In *Human figurations*, P. R. Gleichmann, J. Goudsblom, H. Korte (eds), 110–26. Amsterdam: Amsterdams Sociologisch Tijdschrift.

Wright, E. O. 1985. *Classes*. London: Verso.

Index

Printed and bound by CPI Group (UK) Ltd, Croydon, CR0 4YY

23/10/2024

01777665-0004